THE 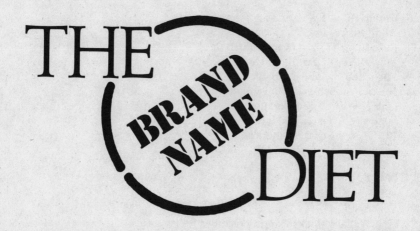 DIET

Leslie-Jane Maynard

A WALLABY BOOK
Published by Simon & Schuster
New York

Published by Wallaby Books
A Simon & Schuster Division of
Gulf & Western Corporation
Simon & Schuster Building
1230 Avenue of the Americas
New York, New York 10020

WALLABY and colophon are registered trademarks
of Simon & Schuster

First Wallaby Books Printing October 1981
10 9 8 7 6 5 4 3 2 1
Manufactured in the United States of America

Library of Congress Cataloging in Publication Data

Maynard, Leslie-Jane.
  The brand name diet.

  "A Wallaby book"
  1. Reducing diets—Recipes.   2. Food industry
and trade—United States.   I. Title.
RM222.2.M394   613.2'5   81-5603
                                      AACR2

ISBN 0-671-41978-1

The information and data contained in this book have been compiled
from authoritative sources. The author does not assume any responsibility
for the products mentioned. The quantity, quality, and ingredients of
these products are subject to change and the reader should be guided
accordingly.

To my best friend Craig

This manuscript would never have made it to press if it had not been for all the caring, hard work and support from Laurie Olsen.

I also want to thank my family for all the times they so joyfully gave assistance.

Contents

Preface

This book is intended not to criticize your former dieting attempts, but to help you to close the door on what has not worked for you and to build a brand new foundation of success.

Like you, I have put myself through almost every conceivable gimmick in dieting. Some were very good, others downright dangerous.

My story is not unique: years of dieting in which weeks of success were followed by months of failure. I was forever in search of the miracle diet that would give me an overnight weight loss. I cannot count how many times I stared at the extravagant claims made in advertisements in newspapers and magazines. Nor can I count the hours I eagerly listened to friends tell me about their latest sensational diet find. Monday was always a good time to start. Better yet, there was the first of the month. That way I was always able to have my "last suppers" and all-out binges before embarking upon what I swore was my last diet attempt.

Let me share some of my experiences. I believe at the conclusion of this preface you will understand why *The Brand Name Diet* came to be.

Eighteen years ago I attended Weight Watchers, a sound nutritional program based on the work of Norman Jolliffe, M.D. At first I was grateful for the guidance and my weight loss from 199 to 135 pounds. Within a few months of attaining my goal, however, I felt trapped rather than secure in the strict regimen. I was angry at the thought of toeing the line to the mandatory five-fish, three-beef and one-liver dinners. Restrictions such as not being allowed to take the bread for breakfast and join it with the bread for lunch to make a sandwich nearly drove me mad. Although an English muffin was about the same in calories as two slices of plain toast, it was considered cheating to make the exchange. String beans cooked one way were permitted for dinner, but, alas, should they be eaten for lunch it was almost a sin. The Weight Watchers magic waned and I abandoned ship. Their program was marvelous, but I could not hack it. I not only regained every pound but added twenty more.

My second hope lay in a physician who promised virtually no hunger with very fast weight loss. Desperate, I was happy to subject myself to diet pills that made me nervous and shaky, diuretics that unnaturally drove fluid out of my body and unnecessary thyroid pills that sped up my burning of calories. The price? Near collapse at the end of a 50-pound weight drop. The result? No longer armed with artificial hunger suppressers and my multicolored capsules that drove away food desires, I climbed on the scale a few months later to find myself where I had started.

My third venture was to visit the office of Dr. Robert C. Atkins. Here I was told of the marvels of eating unlimited meats, eggs and fish and judicious amounts of mayonnaise, butter and oils. All I had to do was remove any and all carbohydrates for one week, said he. I was eager to trade off being hungry for such a small sacrifice. Whenever I wanted to eat, roasted chickens, boiled ham slices, omelets and steaks were permitted in any amount. And indeed, there was a weight loss. In the ensuing weeks tidbits of formerly forbidden carbohydrates were carefully doled out—a small salad, a few green vegetables. I also developed foul-smelling breath (due to being in a state called ketosis), constipation and a slight feeling of nausea. Within a few months, that imprisoned feeling started to emerge once again. I craved to have wine at dinner or an ice-cream cone with my friends or even a small glass of orange juice. His staff firmly vetoed all my requests. I would be throwing off the delicate chemical process and would kill the weight loss. Unable to keep up with the demands of Dr. Atkins's Diet Revolution, I once again bailed out. The outcome? A lesson well learned. The diet did not suit my personal dieting needs. The price? A small weight loss at great sacrifice.

My fourth and final trip down the infernal metal machine known as the scale was one of the best experiences I have ever had in my life. Now armed with knowledge from the above-mentioned dieting failures, some fascinating and solid education in both psychology and nutrition, I carefully planned out a diet that would suit all my wants without sacrificing good physical or mental health. My list of needs looked somewhat like the following:

1. Total flexibility in my eating schedule.
2. Ability to incorporate any and all foods on about 1200 calories per day.
3. A system that would allow me to bank the calories for a sumptuous feast. As an example, I could bring my diet down to 900 calories per day Monday through Friday and have an extra 1500 calories to play with as I saw fit Saturday and Sunday. Weekends were and still are my most playful days on all levels. I needed a joyous food feeling to complement and enhance our dinner parties, social gatherings and movie outings, to keep me company getting lost in a terrific novel and curling up with the Sunday *New York Times*.
4. A method that would allow me to instantly forgive myself should I deviate from my food plan.

At first, as I reviewed my notes, I thought the project would be an impossibility. However, as I tackled each area it soon became apparent that indeed a fabulous diet was emerging. I felt like a mad food scientist plowing through the *Composition of Foods Agriculture Handbook No. 8.* This nifty publication from the United States Department of Agriculture (USDA) told of magical exchanges, substitutions and trade-offs that could be made by choosing a variety of foods. Although I was not smitten by cooked roasted muskrat yielding 153 calories for 3½ ounces versus opossum having 221 calories, it quickly became apparent that 93 calories and 17.3 grams of protein for 3½ ounces of succulent steamed crabmeat was a superb choice over smoked eel for 330 calories at 18.6 grams of protein!!

Hundreds upon hundreds of my favorite foods were now clearly within my reach. But oh how I longed for an Oreo cookie or a Hershey bar. They were nowhere to be found in my treasured USDA reference. And so, I scoured through many a calorie-counting book, wrote directly to food companies and marched up and down the aisles of supermarkets checking can after box after package for nutritional data. Soon Pillsbury, General Foods, Nabisco, McDonald's, Carvel, Sealtest and many more companies sent envelopes which poured out of my mailbox week by week. All my questions were answered. I felt like a composer. With all these marvelous "food notes," I started to create my "Maynard Fifth Symphony Diet." Making additions to my symphony was as easy as pie. I then played my composition for a few weeks and to my total amazement dropped about 17 pounds in two months while feasting.

This last venture ended in a secure, contented and fulfilled 135-pound body. That was eight years ago. To this day my love affair with my diet continues.

Introduction

The word *diet* usually conjures up the following feelings in our minds: deprivation, punishment, imprisonment and anger.

The diet that was famous in 1979 planned your every meal Monday morning through Sunday night. Prior to that, there was the very popular diet which restricted your carbohydrate intake. In the past we have also seen a high-protein diet accompanied by countless glasses of water, not to mention the outrageous diet which took food away entirely and replaced it with liquid protein. Countless weight-watching organizations have sprung up throughout our country in the last thirty years with sound low-calorie diets—and of course there is the well-known self-help group which follows some of the guidelines of Alcoholics Anonymous.

Diets come and go. Fad foods spring up one day and fade out the next. New theories are born and laid to rest as quickly as they are developed. Why? A theory is based on an accumulation of ideas, facts, conjectures and opinions. But a fact is based on proven data. For instance, it is a fact that if you lower your weekly caloric intake by 3500 calories you will lose 1 pound of body fat. It is also a fact that if you expend 3500 calories worth of energy over and beyond your daily caloric requirement you will also lose 1 pound of body fat. But it is a theory that the best way to burn those 3500 calories is by eating grapefruit.

All of the above brings me to the following. The Brand Name Diet is based on facts, not opinions—facts that have been gathered for you from the various food companies, or that are found in USDA *Composition of Foods Handbook No. 8*. Using these facts, I have devised a food plan that will allow you to decide how, when, and what you want to eat.

It is my theory that this book will work only for the person who is interested in taking control and making decisions. I do not believe that my work will serve for those people who are looking for an authoritarian leadership. My beliefs are based on the fact that most people want to be free. Whether in government, lifestyle or religion, the quest for freedom has always been a strong motivation. You as an individual are therefore entitled to make up your food plan according to your total needs.

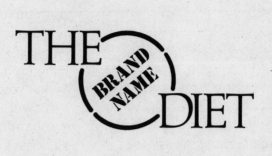
THE BRAND NAME DIET

I

Anatomy of the Supermarket

Most authors who formulate diets are concerned with what food you put in your mouth. You are given techniques on cooking, preparing and serving. I find the most neglected part of slimming (as they call dieting in England) is *shopping*. This is precisely what The Brand Name Diet concerns itself with. Let's go on a tour in a typical market.

Walking through a supermarket is much like looking at a set designed for a play. The supermarket owner wants you to buy and the supermarket designer draws you into the plot.

SCENE I

We take a cart. Usually the first aisle we come to is abundant with produce, that is, fruits and vegetables. Carefully filed in among the greens are luscious-looking bottles of salad dressings, not to mention the new potato toppings and an assortment of nuts. Often a good produce manager will sprinkle water over the in-store garden to give it that just-picked look. It also keeps everything crunchy and fresh. It's inviting, and we feel compelled to buy something even though we may not really need it.

SCENE II

We turn our cart toward the back of the store and are now greeted with meats, poultry, sausages, fish, etc., in a striking array of colors. Often the lighting system used over the meat counters has a color-enhancement feature which makes the red appear redder. We have been indoctrinated to think that red meat is healthy for us, giving us vim and vigor.

The packaged deli meat and frankfurters follow. Here the assortment can boggle the imagination!

SCENE III

The delicatessen counter usually follows along the back wall. Again, countless varieties of ham, bolognas, cheeses, rolls, smoked fish, assorted breads, salads and candies beckon us. A savvy deli manager knows that samplings of various items will increase sales! *And our girth!*

SCENE IV

Next we turn the cart down the dairy aisle. Here the land of every conceivable milk product, from creams to yogurts to cheeses to eggs to puddings to dips, etc., enthralls us. There are so many types of American cheese, American processed cheese and American processed cheese food that the confusion alone can keep us a captive buyer. I sometimes think that the more we stand there the more we buy.

SCENE V

On to other aisles. Bakery goods summon us to attractive cellophane wrappings and boxed confections. Muffins look as though we must take them home. Breadsticks incite dreams of parties; loaves of bread, images of hearty sandwiches; and cakes, fantasies of joyful celebrations! On to the cracker and cookie aisle—a pièce de résistance. Boxes upon boxes picture mouthwatering experiences. Nabisco has done a superb job of luring the buyer to its corner. The lifelike pictures on the boxes are enough to start activating anyone's salivary glands! The candy and cereal sections are enough to send someone to Harvard, Princeton or Yale to study a postgraduate course in selection. Phrases such as "sound bodies" and "fresh-start mornings" blare at us to buy, buy, buy!

Frozen Foodland is our next stop. Here major countries are presented in full food splendor—China, Italy, France, Mexico and Israel! Plain frozen vegetables are huddled in a corner to make room for hearty, "man-sized" entrees, specialties for one or two, mini-desserts and banquet-sized feasts for a crowd. Creamed this and stuffed that, not to mention au gratin, fried and baked! Ice creams? You jest! Which color, flavor or size, not to mention price range? People have been known to develop frostbite just rummaging through the various cartons of frozen delights.

Of course, I have not covered the entire market. My point was only to show you how careful merchandising can make you prey to overbuying or buying things that may not be good for you. Here are some hints that I think may be valuable to you.

1. Next time you go to your supermarket, plan on its being solely a look-see tour without actually shopping for any-

thing. Try to figure out why you want to purchase a certain product. Is it because it was advertised as the latest thing to buy? Was it beautifully displayed in a magazine which bore a 10-cents-off coupon? Is it currently on special at a reduced price? Or is it simply an item that you like and have repeatedly been buying? Finding out why you do something can be the key to understanding some of your shopping behavior.

2. Are you usually hungry at the time you do your shopping? The consensus among food psychologists is that to shop on an empty stomach is to ask for trouble. I heartily concur. Therefore, make sure that the next time you set out to market you do so with a full tummy.

3. Do you shop with a list in hand? Many times people think that they will remember exactly what they need once they arrive at the market. I have found that most times often-needed items are forgotten and many non-needed ones are added. Always take a home inventory of your food stock and march to the supermarket armed with your list!

4. Who is with you at the time that you are doing your shopping? Cranky and tired children are not good shopping companions—especially when they scream for this or that and you succumb to buying something just to keep them quiet. If the children are tired, make arrangements to have a baby-sitter and shop alone!

5. Are you under stress at the time you usually shop for food? You may be distracted by problems and not able to concentrate on what you are doing. This can lead to indiscriminate grabbing of items. If you are feeling depressed or sorry for yourself you might be tempted to buy something to heal your emotional wounds. I suggest that shopping for food be as technical an experience as possible. Emotions should not have an influence over your choices.

In closing this chapter, I want to emphasize that the market need not be a place of diet destruction. Rather it should and can be a place of sound diet construction. In the next chapter we will get to the "meat" of this book.

II

Caveat Emptor—
Buyer Beware

To show you that I am not suffering from delusions of diet grandeur, I shall attempt to amaze and captivate you with the following almost-humorous comparisons for a one-day diet.

My work here is solely devoted to enhancement of your shopping knowledge. For it is through your awareness that you will be able to make appropriate decisions.

Let us now look at two choices of diets. You can then decide for yourself.

HIGH- AND LOW-CALORIE SUPERMARKET CHOICES

In order for you to understand why careful shopping for food is so crucial to your diet, I have given comparisons in the chart below.

NOTE: Basically both diets are the same in choices. The differences are brand names and some amounts.

THE BRAND NAME DIET

THE HIGH-CALORIE MENU

Breakfast

2	slices Pepperidge Farm wheat bread	180
2	tsps. Smucker's strawberry jam	36
½	cup Borden creamed cottage cheese	120
6	oz. Ocean Spray Cranberry Juice Cocktail	108
	TOTAL	444

Lunch

	assorted raw vegetables: ½ cup carrots, 4 celery stalks, 1 cucumber, 1 cup cauliflower	100
1	8-oz. container Dannon strawberry yogurt	260
	TOTAL	360

Dinner

1	9-oz. portion of Gorton's fillet of sole entree	400
1	large assorted lettuce salad with 2 Tbsp. Good Seasons Thousand Island Thick 'n Creamy dressing	173
½	cup Birds Eye frozen mixed Vegetable Jubilee in cream sauce	138
1	medium baked potato with 1 tablespoon Breakstone butter	192
1	cup Diet Delight unpeeled halved apricots, blue label	120
½	cup vanilla Häagen-Dazs ice cream	267
	TOTAL	1,290

THE LOW-CALORIE MENU

Breakfast

2	slices Pepperidge Farm whole wheat bread	70
2	tsps. Smucker's Low Sugar Strawberry spread	16
½	cup Borden Lite-line low-fat cottage cheese	90
6	oz. low-calorie Ocean Spray cranberry juice	39
	TOTAL	215

Lunch

	assorted raw vegetables: ½ cup carrots, 4 celery stalks, 1 cucumber, 1 cup cauliflower	100
1	8-oz. container Sweet 'n Low strawberry yogurt	150
	TOTAL	250

Dinner

1	6-oz. portion of Gorton's Cod in Cheese Sauce	180
1	large assorted lettuce salad with 2 Tbsp. Kraft low-calorie Thousand Island dressing	83
½	cup Green Giant mixed frozen vegetables in butter sauce	67
1	medium baked potato with Breakstone whipped butter	159
1	cup Diet Delight unpeeled halved apricots, green label	70
½	cup Sealtest Light n' Lively vanilla ice cream	100
	TOTAL	659

Snack			Snack		
1	wedge Laughing Cow (la vache qui rit) cheese	74	1	wedge reduced-calorie Laughing Cow (la vache qui rit) cheese	35
5	Nabisco mister salty 3-ring pretzels	60	30	Nabisco mister salty Veri-Thin Pretzel Sticks	35
6	fl. oz. Dr Pepper soda	71	6	fl. oz. Sugar Free Dr Pepper soda	2
TOTAL		205	TOTAL		72
GRAND TOTAL FOR THE DAY:		**2,299**	GRAND TOTAL FOR THE DAY:		**1,196**

As you can see from the above, the low-calorie versions save you more than one-half the calories, but give you about equal the taste, portion and nutritional value. The only thing you lose is weight!

My point has been made: *Selection* of foods is the key to weight control. In the following chapter we will work together on the diet itself. But first I want to point out some unbelievable examples in this fascinating sample diet you have just read.

Note that cottage cheese is still basically cottage cheese, but by lowering the fat content there's a drop of 30 calories. The same applies to the bread, the strawberry spread and jam, and the Ocean spray cranberry juice. In other words, the breakfast really did not consist of trading off bread for melba toast and strawberry jam for two fresh strawberries, or cottage cheese for egg whites and cranberry juice for water. The selections were different, but the foods ostensibly stayed the same.

The same goes for the diet throughout this book. At dinner you will notice that five Nabisco Triscuit wafers for 110 calories have been replaced by 5 Nabisco wheat thins for 45 calories. You are very justified if you say, "Well, the Triscuit wafer is larger than the wheat thins." True, you cannot have everything that you want. But by decalorizing the choices, you can lose weight and still eat the foods that taste good to you!

I find the most fascinating part of this one-day romp with food to be the snack . . . with one wedge of Laughing Cow Cheese at 74 calories versus one wedge of reduced-calorie Laughing Cow Cheese at 35 calories. Need I say more about having five Nabisco mister salty 3-Ring Pretzels for 60 calories when you can munch on thirty Nabisco mister salty Veri-Thin Pretzel Sticks for almost half the calories?

These are just a few samples of the delights that await you in the ensuing pages. I hope I have sufficiently whetted your appetite for what is to become a feast with weight loss. *But*, before we get to the diet itself, I must include a very small chapter that has to do with your health. Read on, MacDuff!

III

A Toast to Your Health

Your health is your most valuable physical asset. I may be bold in my approach to dieting, but I want you to know that I am highly conservative in my approach to well-being. The Brand Name Diet, as you will see, does contain foods that heretofore no nutritionist would basically think sound to include. Doughnuts, chocolates, candies, fast foods, etc., have never really been thought healthy enough to include in a weight-reduction program. I believe that if these foods are abused, ill health may set in. Since you will always have to make the decisions about which foods you *are* going to choose from The Brand Name Diet, I think it is imperative for me to share with you the following list of nutrients, why they are needed, and their food sources. Again, this is an adult and independent approach in dieting. I simply give you the information and you take on the responsibility of making the appropriate decisions.

Technically, since you are given the choice to make choices, under "Protein" you might decide to only use peanut butter or under "Carbohydrates" to only use jam, or under "Fats" to concentrate on chocolate candies. This kind of attitude would of course be preposterous. My intention —and I reiterate, this has to do with your health—is to show you that you can indeed safely include those "forbidden foods," but that you must not abuse them. I can impart the knowledge, but only you have the power to put the knowledge to work. A wide variety of choices will help you ensure a proper balance of nutrients. Your physician should recommend the appropriate multi-vitamin with minerals to supplement your diet.

Now let us look at the following:

NUTRIENT AND WHY IT IS NEEDED	FOOD SOURCES
1. Protein Promotes growth and the repair of body tissues; supplies energy and helps to fight infections; forms a very important part of your blood and enzymes. In addition, it helps your hormones regulate your body functions.	Lean meats, poultry, fish, shellfish, eggs, milk, cheese. Next best are the vegetable proteins such as dried beans and peas, nuts, peanut butter, bread, cereals, and wheat germ. If served with a complementary animal protein or in complementary pairs with foods such as cheese, the combined protein value is high.
2. Carbohydrates (Sugars and starches) Help save protein for body building and repair; necessary for bulk and proper elimination. In addition, supply energy.	Breads, cereals, grits, corn, rice, potatoes, the macaroni and noodle families, fruits, vegetables, sugar, honey, syrup, jam, jelly.
3. Fats Supply concentrated energy; help the body to use other nutrients; help maintain body temperature; lubricate the intestinal tract.	Butter, margarine, whole milk, ice cream, cheese, egg yolk, shortening, chocolate, pies (e.g., coconut cream), puddings, salad oils.

4. Calcium

Builds sturdy bones and teeth; helps the blood's clotting mechanism; helps heart, muscles and nerves function properly; also aids in healing of wounds and helps to fight off infections.

Milk, ice cream, cheese, cottage cheese, kale, collards, turnip greens, salmons, sardines.

5. Phosphorus

Essential (along with calcium) for teeth and bones; aids fat to do its job in your body; in addition, helps the enzymes that are used in energy metabolism.

Milk, ice cream, cheese, meat, poultry, whole grain cereals, dried beans and peas, fish, nuts.

6. Magnesium

An absolute for strong bones and teeth; aids in the transmitting of nerve impulses; helps muscle contraction.

Cereals, dried beans, meats, milk, whole grains, egg yolks, green vegetables, nuts.

7. Iron

Necessary to form hemoglobin (the red substance in your blood which carries the oxygen from your lungs to your body cells.)

Liver, kidneys, oysters, lean meats, egg yolk, clams, whole-grain and enriched cereals, dried beans, raisins, dark green leafy vegetables.

8. Iodine

Helps your thyroid gland to work properly in regulating your energy.

Iodized salt, saltwater fish and shellfish, mushrooms.

9. Sodium

Preserves the water balance in your body.

Salt, cured meat, fish, eggs, olives, cheese.

10. Potassium

Helps to keep nerves and muscles healthy; in addition, maintains the body's fluid balance.

Oranges, bananas, potatoes (with peel), whole grains, green leafy vegetables.

11. Vitamin A
Helps to maintain your eyesight, especially under dim lighting; aids in the growth of healthy skin, bones and teeth; helps to promote growth and resist infection.

Liver, broccoli, turnips, carrots, pumpkin, sweet potatoes, winter squash, apricots, butter, fortified margarine, egg yolk, fish-liver oils, cantaloupe.

12. Vitamin D
Helps your body to use both calcium and phosphorus, which are needed to build strong bones and teeth.

Fortified milk, fish-liver oils, egg yolk, liver, salmon, tuna. Direct sunlight also produces Vitamin D.

13. Vitamin E
Although its function is not clearly understood, it is thought to help in the formation of red blood cells, muscle and other tissue.

Wheat-germ oil, salad oils, green leafy vegetables, nuts, dried beans and peas, margarine.

14. Vitamin K
Helps to promote normal blood clotting.

Green leafy vegetables, cauliflower, egg yolk, liver, soybean oil.

15. Thiamine (Vitamin B$_1$)
Helps your body cells to obtain energy from food; aids in keeping your nerves healthy; in addition, promotes good appetite and digestion.

Pork, lean meats, poultry, fish, liver, dried beans and peas, egg yolk, whole-grain and enriched cereals and breads, soybeans.

16. Riboflavin (Vitamin B$_2$)
Helps the body to use proteins, fats and carbohydrates, which are needed for energy and for building tissues; promotes a radiant-looking skin and aids in the maintenance of eyesight.

Milk, cheese, liver, kidneys, eggs, green leafy vegetables, enriched cereals and breads.

17. Niacin
Required for a healthy nervous system, digestive tract and skin, in addition, aids energy production in cells.

Lean meats, poultry, fish, varied packaged meats, dark green leafy vegetables, whole-grain and enriched cereals and breads, peanuts, wheat germ.

18. Vitamin B$_6$

Aids the body to use the intake of protein and also helps to maintain a normal hemoglobin level in the blood.

Meats, wheat germ, liver, whole-grain cereals, soybeans, kidneys, peanuts.

19. Vitamin B$_{12}$

A necessity for the production of red blood cells and for building new proteins in your body.

Meats, liver, kidneys, fish, eggs, milk, cheese.

20. Vitamin C (Ascorbic Acid)

Aids in the building of the materials that hold cells together; vital in helping wounds to heal and to resist infection. Also needed for maintaining healthy teeth, gums, and blood vessels.

Citrus fruits, strawberries, cantaloupes, tomatoes, potatoes, brussels sprouts, raw cabbage, broccoli, green and sweet red peppers.

21. Folic Acid

Helps to maintain a normal red blood cell count; required for a healthy nervous system and essential in the formation of certain body proteins and genetic materials in the cell nucleus.

Green leafy vegetables, especially raw spinach, lean beef and veal, liver, citrus fruits, soybeans and nuts.

To continue the list with items such as zinc, biotin, copper, silicon, fluorine and many more would require almost another book. Check your library for a good reference source if you are interested. There are several books by Barbara Kraus that provide excellent nutritional information: *The Barbara Kraus Dictionary of Protein, The Barbara Kraus Guide to Fiber in Foods,* and *The Barbara Kraus 1980 Carbohydrate Guide to Brand Names and Basic Foods.* Also you might consult The United States Department of Agriculture Yearbook 1979, *What's to Eat?*

Now I believe we are ready for the grand diet experience!

As with any and all diets, consult with your physician first before embarking on The Brand Name Diet.

IV

The Brand Name Diet

The Brand Name Diet is written for a twenty-four hour period. In other words, you will have the freedom to decide for yourself *when* you are going to eat; there are no required meal plans. You will also have the freedom to decide for yourself *what* you are going to eat; there are no required foods.

Everything has been calculated for you. No more calorie charts, no more counting carbohydrate grams, no more guessing, no more frustration!!!

Remember: You may eat as many times as you wish during a twenty-four-hour period, and you may choose exactly what appeals to you for that time. You do not have to eat if you are not hungry, and you may eat if you are. What could be better than total *freedom?!!!*

The Brand Name Diet is based on the principle of a wide variety of choices. Everyday, you will be able to make your selections from the following twelve categories:

① The Bakery, Cereal Bowl & Grain Bin
② The Milk Barn & The Ice-Cream Parlor
③ The Vegetable Patch, The Fruit Stand & The Dried Bean Sack
④ The Butcher Block & The Fisherman's Net
⑤ The Soup Tureen & The Juice Pitcher
⑥ The Hen's Nest, The Cheese Shed & The Deli
⑦ The Tiny Items That Make a Big Sensation & The Pub
⑧ The Salad Bowl
⑨ The Salad Dressing, Butter & Bacon Corner
⑩ To Your Heart's Content
⑪ The International Buffet
⑫ How to Eat at McDonald's, Burger King, Arthur Treacher's, Etc.

As you browse through The Brand Name Diet you may feel overwhelmed because there are so many choices. Remember! The numerous choices are part of the magic and freedom this diet offers.

You may have to do some daily homework in order to become skilled at menu planning. However, you can personalize the diet and simplify preparing your shopping list by circling the choices you prefer and crossing out those you never select.

Remember to shop carefully! Food manufacturers frequently market different products under similar names: Beef Noodle soup is not the same as Hearty Beef with Noodles, and the calorie differences may be extreme.

How to Follow *The Brand Name Diet*

In the course of each twenty-four hour period, *The Brand Name Diet* allows you to select a specified number of choices, divided in a variety of ways, from each of the twelve categories.

You may find it difficult to remember how much you are entitled to eat from each category and how much you have already eaten. The chart on page 34 solves this problem by allowing you to keep track of what you have eaten and what you may eat. The number and name of each category is followed by its corresponding number of choices. Each time you use a choice, simply cross it out.

For instance, there are two choices (or four halves) in ③ The Vegetable Patch, The Fruit Stand & The Dried Bean Sack. Each time you use up a choice simply put a slash through it.

Example: If you've already eaten 1 cup blueberries and 1½ medium tomatoes, your chart should read ~~half~~, ~~half~~, ~~half~~, half, since you used one choice (half + half) with the blueberries and half a choice with the tomatoes. By using the chart, you can clearly see the choices you have used and the choices you have left to use.

Hint: Make copies of the chart for daily use.

Daily Inventory

① The Bakery, Cereal Bowl &
Grain Bin · CHOICES: half + half

② The Milk Barn & The Ice
Cream Parlor · CHOICES: half + half

③ The Vegetable Patch, the
Fruit Stand & the Dried Bean
Sack · CHOICES: half + half + half + half

④ The Butcher Block & The
Fisherman's Net · CHOICES: half + half

⑤ The Soup Tureen & the Juice
Pitcher · CHOICES: one (cannot be divided)

⑥ The Hen's Nest, The cheese
Shed & The Deli · CHOICES: half + half

⑦ The Tiny Items That Make a
Big Sensation & the Pub · CHOICES: half + half + half + half

⑧ The Salad Bowl · CHOICES: unlimited

⑨ The Salad Dressing, Butter &
Bacon Corner · CHOICES: half + half

⑩ To Your Heart's Content · CHOICES: unlimited

⑪ The International Buffet · CHOICES: combination

⑫ How to Eat at McDonald's,
Burger King, Arthur
Treacher's, Etc. · CHOICES: combination

Remember: one choice = half + half
two choices = half + half + half + half

SAMPLE DAILY MENU

Now that you have seen how to plan your OWN menu, here is a sample of how a day might shape up:

BREAKFAST

2 slices whole wheat Pepperidge Farm thin sliced bread
    (half from ① The Bakery, Cereal Bowl & Grain Bin)
AND

8 oz. tomato juice
    (one from ⑤ The Soup Tureen & The Juice Pitcher)
AND

1 slice Lite-line cheese
    (half from ⑥ The Hen's Nest, The Cheese Shed & The Deli)
AND

Beverage of your choice
    (unlimited from ⑩ To Your Heart's Content)

SNACK

1 large carrot
    (half from ③ The Vegetable Patch, The Fruit Stand & The Dried Bean Sack

LUNCH

2½ slices Oscar Mayer Smoked Cooked Ham
    (half from ⑥ The Hen's Nest, The Cheese Shed & The Deli)
AND

2 sesame Stella D'Oro bread sticks
    (half from ① The Bakery, Cereal Bowl & Grain Bin)
AND

Salad of your choice
   (unlimited from ⑧ The Salad Bowl
                                    AND
1 tablespoon Kraft Thousand Island dressing
   (half from ⑨ The Salad Dressing, Butter & Bacon
   Corner)
                                    AND
½ large grapefruit
   (half from ③ The Vegetable Patch, The Fruit Stand &
   The Dried Bean Sack)

SNACK

35 Nabisco mister salty Veri-Thin Pretzel sticks
   (half from ⑦ The Tiny Items That Make a Big Sensation
   & The Pub)

DINNER

8 medium raw clams on the half shell
   (half from ④ The Butcher Block & The Fisherman's Net)
                                    AND
5 oz. steamed lobster
   (half from ④ The Butcher Block & The Fisherman's Net)
                                    AND
½ medium baked potato
   (half from ③ The Vegetable Patch, The Fruit Stand &
   The Dried Bean Sack)
                                    AND
1 tablespoon sour cream
   (half from ⑦ The Tiny Items That Make a Big Sensation
   & The Pub)
                                    AND

Salad of your choice
  (unlimited from ⑧ The Salad Bowl)
                        AND
1 tablespoon Kraft imitation mayonnaise
  (half from ⑨ The Salad Dressing, Butter & Bacon
  Corner)
                        AND
Beverage of your choice
  (unlimited from ⑩ To Your Heart's Content)
                        AND
serving of Orange dietetic gelatin
  (unlimited from ⑩ To Your Heart's Content)
                        AND

SNACK

½ cup chocolate ice milk such as Light n' Lively
  (one from ② The Milk Barn & The Ice Cream Parlor)
                        AND
½ medium banana
  (half from ③ The Vegetable Patch, The Fruit Stand &
  The Dried Bean Sack)
                        AND
1 tablespoon Hershey's chocolate syrup
  (half from ⑦ The Tiny Items That Make a Big Sensation
  & The Pub)
                        AND
2 tablespoons Cool Whip topping
  (half from ⑦ The Tiny Items That Make a Big Sensation
  & The Pub)

An incredible banana split!

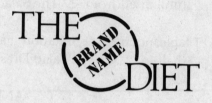

The Bakery, Cereal Bowl & Grain Bin

Follow these instructions for enjoying The Bakery, Cereal Bowl & Grain Bin. (Where there is no brand name for an item, it is always *any brand*.) There are numerous groups from which you may choose your one choice for the day and several ways you can treat this choice:

A. You may pick *one* choice

   or

B. You may pick *two* choices and simply divide the amount of each choice in *half*.

THE BAKERY

THE BREAD BASKET

2 slices any kind presliced bread
   (an average slice is about 1 ounce)
5 slices Thomas' Glutogen Gluten bread
4 slices Pepperidge Farm thin slice, any variety

1 English Muffin, plain
1 bagel, Lender's frozen pre-sliced plain, egg or onion
1 hamburger roll
1 frankfurter roll
1 hard roll, deli type
1 onion roll
1 pita (pocket bread of the Middle East), any brand, 160
   calories maximum

THE BUN WARMER

Pepperidge Farm

3 Brown & Serve rolls
5 Party Pan rolls
3 Finger rolls, sesame or poppy

Pillsbury

2 Hungry Jack extra light biscuits
2 Parkerhouse rolls

THE WAFFLE IRON

1 jumbo frozen Aunt Jemina or Downyflake Waffle
1 frozen Eggo waffle, any variety

THE POP-UP TOASTER

4 Thomas' Toast-r-Cake, any variety

THE DOUGHNUT SHOP

1 donut, any brand, plain cake type without icing or filling
1 frozen Morton glazed donut (from 9⅛-oz. box)
1 yeast-raised plain donut—Dunkin' Donuts Shops
6 yeast-raised plain Munchkins—Dunkin' Donuts Shops

THE CAKE SERVER

Drake's

1 Drake's Yankee Doodle
1 Drake's plain pound cake (1.6 oz., individually wrapped slice)
1 (1.1-oz.) Drake's Coffee Cake Jr.
1 (1.1-oz.) piece Drake's Dozy Oats
1 Hostess orange cupcake
1 lemon creme-filled or vanilla cream-filled Tastycake cupcake
1 *sliver* of any cake should there be a special occasion where you cannot control the choice
1 Sara Lee individually frozen crumb cake

THE COOKIE JAR

Nabisco

1 dozen Vanilla Snaps
6 Brown Edge Wafers
1 dozen Barnum's Animal Crackers
8 Chocolate Snaps
10 Ginger Zu-Zu Snaps
10 Lemon Snaps
8 Social Tea Biscuits
8 Nilla Wafers

Stella D'Oro

4 Anisette Toast
4 Egg Biscuits (Jumbo), dietetic
20 Dietetic Kichel
80 Royal Nuggets, dietetic

THE CRACKER BARREL

15 Old London Melba Toast Rounds, any variety
50 Oyster Crackers
12 Saltine Cracker squares

Nabisco

30 Cheese Nips
150 YES!! 150 Nabisco mister salty Veri-Thin Pretzel Sticks
80 Chipsters
15 Sociables
18 wheat thins

Pepperidge Farm

50 Goldfish, any variety

General Mills

40 Whistles

THE BREAD STICK JAR

4 sesame Stella D'Oro bread sticks
4 plain Stella D'Oro bread sticks
4 onion flavored Stella D'Oro bread sticks

STUFFING, CRUMBS & SUCH

8 tablespoons bread crumbs
½ cup chicken, pork or cornbread Stove Top stuffing mix,
    prepared as package directs
¾ cup Pepperidge Farm Stuffing Bread Cubes
¾ cup Pepperidge Farm Corn Bread Stuffing
¾ cup Pepperidge Farm Herb Seasoned Bread Stuffing

THE BRAND NAME DIET

1 ounce Pepperidge Farm Onion & Garlic Croutons
1 ounce Pepperidge Farm Seasoned Croutons with Herbs
  and Cheese
1 ounce Pepperidge Farm Cheese & Garlic Croutons
1 ounce Pepperidge Farm Sour Cream & Chive Croutons
1 ounce Pepperidge Farm Cheddar & Romano Cheese
  Croutons

THE MATZO BASKET

1 sheet matzo, any variety
15 Goodman's Diet-10's
12 Manischewitz Tams Tams, any variety
20 Manischewitz Matzo Cracker Miniatures

THE CEREAL BOWL

1¼ cups 40% Bran Flakes
1½ cups Cheerios
1½ cups Corn Chex
½ cup Kellogg's Concentrate
1½ cups Corn Flakes
⅓ cup Post Grape-Nuts
1 cup Post Grape-Nuts Flakes
1 cup Quaker Life
1½ cups Kellogg's Product 19
3 cups Quaker puffed rice
4 cups Quaker puffed wheat
1½ cups Rice Krispies
2 Nabisco Shredded Wheat Biscuits
1 cup Nabisco Spoon Size Shredded Wheat
1¾ cups Kellogg's Special K
1½ cups Total

1½ cups Wheaties
⅓ cup plain wheat germ

THE STEAMING CEREAL BOWL

4 tablespoons dry Nabisco Cream of Wheat, instant, quick
  or regular
1 cup cooked farina
1 cup cooked hominy grits
¼ cup uncooked 30-second Maypo
1 cup cooked oatmeal
¼ cup uncooked Wheatena

THE GRAIN & PASTA BIN

1 cup tender cooked spaghetti or macaroni
(14 to 20 minutes cooking time)
¾ cup cooked noodles
⅔ cup white or brown rice
½ cup any cooked rice mix (other than Chinese fried rice)

The Milk Barn &
The Ice-Cream Parlor

Follow these instructions for enjoying The Milk Barn & The
Ice Cream Parlor. (Where there is no brand name for an
item, it is always *any brand*.) There are numerous groups
from which you may select your one choice for the day and
several ways you can treat this choice.

THE BRAND NAME DIET

A. You may pick *one* choice
 or
B. You may pick *two* choices and simply divide the amount
of each choice in *half.*

THE MILK BARN

12 oz. modified skimmed milk
8 oz. 99% fat-free skimmed milk
8 oz. buttermilk with 1% or less butterfat
6 oz. whole milk
2 envelopes Alba 66, any flavor
1 8-oz. container of plain yogurt (made from partially
 skimmed milk)
½ cup any flavor D-Zerta pudding prepared with skimmed
 milk
1 8-oz. container any flavor Sweet n' Low yogurt

THE ICE-CREAM PARLOR

1 3-oz. cup of any flavor Sealtest ice cream
1 3-oz. cup of vanilla or chocolate Dairy Queen soft ice
 cream
1 Creamsicle
1 3-oz. cup vanilla or chocolate Good Humor ice cream
1 Danny (Dannon) frozen yogurt on a stick, any flavor
 (chocolate coated)
2 3-oz. cups of any flavor Carvel Thinny Thin
½ cup any flavor ice milk, such as Light n' Lively
1 7-oz. cup Weight Watchers Frosted Treat Frozen Desert
2 plain vanilla Danny yogurt on a stick
1 serving (5 fl. oz.) Weight Watchers Snack Cups, any
 flavor

1 small Dairy Queen soft ice cream, plain cone
1 3-fl. oz. bar Weight Watchers Chocolate Treat

The Vegetable Patch, The Fruit Stand & The Dried Bean Sack

This section may be a new world of food for you. It's nutritionally good for you and it will help you to lose weight.

Follow these instructions for enjoying The Vegetable Patch, The Fruit Stand & The Dried Bean Sack. There are numerous groups from which you may select your two choices for the day and several ways you can treat these choices.

A. You may pick the same choice *twice*
    or
B. You may pick *two* different choices
    or
C. You may pick *four* different choices by dividing the amount of each choice in *half*.

It's really very easy once you get into the swing of it. Just to give you an idea:

What do you think of being able to have 2 medium potatoes or 1 cup cooked and drained lentils by selecting suggestion A? *Freedom!!!*

What do you think of being able to have 1 medium ear of corn *and* 1 medium potato by selecting suggestion B? *Freedom!!!*

What do you think of being able to have half a medium
potato *and* 1¼ cups of green beans *and* ½ large grapefruit
and an 8-oz. glass of tomato juice by selecting suggestion
C? *Freedom!!!*

The mixing and matching is endless. You have the freedom to make your own decisions and the freedom to follow
your own desires. Have fun exploring! The following choices
may be eaten *raw* or *cooked*. You can select from *fresh, frozen*
or *canned*. The vegetables should not be purchased in
creamed or buttered sauces or be sweet-and-sour pickled—
unless noted.

THE VEGETABLE PATCH

¼ of a medium avocado
1 large artichoke
20 artichoke hearts or 1½ boxes frozen artichoke hearts
35 asparagus spears
2½ cups green or wax beans
½ cup lima beans
1½ cups bamboo shoots
2½ cups bean sprouts
1½ cups beets
4 cups beet greens
2½ cups broccoli
1 cup brussels sprouts
3½ cups any kind of cabbage
4 large carrots or 2 cups
3 cups cauliflower
3 cups Swiss chard
½ cup Chinese water chestnuts
2 cups collards

Vegetable Patch, Fruit Stand & Dried Bean Sack

1 medium ear of corn
½ cup corn kernels
½ cup creamed corn
4 cups ready-to-eat popped corn, prepared without fat
3 large cucumbers
2½ cups eggplant
1½ cups kale
1½ cups kohlrabi
5 cups mushrooms
32 pods okra or 2 cups
2 medium onions
¾ cup parsnips
¾ cup peas
10 frozen french fried potatoes, prepared without any
    additional fat
8 green or 5 red peppers
6 large pickles or 12 medium of any kind other than sweet
1 medium potato, or 1 tiny sweet potato or yam
1 cup pumpkin, plain
3 cups sauerkraut
½ cup frozen chopped creamed spinach, Seabrook Farms
5 cups raw spinach, fresh or 1½ 9-oz. boxes of frozen
    spinach (not creamed), or 2 cups canned spinach
1¼ cup acorn squash
1 cup butternut squash
1 cup hubbard squash
3 cups any summer squash
½ cup succotash
3 medium tomatoes
3 stewed tomatoes
1 cup tomato puree
1 cup canned tomato sauce
1 8-oz. can of Contadina tomato sauce

1 8-oz. can of Hunt's Tomato Sauce with Mushrooms
½ cup tomato paste
2 cups turnips
2½ cups turnip greens
4 cups La Choy Chinese canned mixed vegetables
1 cup mixed vegetables

THE FRUIT STAND

Important note: The following choices may be eaten *raw* or *cooked*. You may select from *frozen, fresh* or *canned*.

Frozen and canned fruits: In measuring out fruits, use as little syrup as possible.

1 medium apple
1 cup unsweetened Mott's applesauce
½ cup sweetened applesauce
5 apricots
1 cup Diet Delight (green label) apricots
½ cup heavy-syrup apricots
1 medium banana
1 cup fresh blackberries
1 cup blueberries
¾ cup diet-pack cherries (without liquid)
½ cup heavy-syrup cherries
2 cups fresh cranberries
3 tablespoons regular canned cranberry sauce, whole or jellied
¾ cup diet-pack fruit cocktail (without liquid)
½ cup heavy-syrup fruit cocktail
5 average-size dates
1 cup grapes
1 large grapefruit

¾ cup diet-pack grapefruit sections (without liquid)
½ cup heavy-syrup grapefruit sections
1 medium cantaloupe
2 cups cubed honeydew melon
¾ cup frozen melon balls in regular syrup
1 cup diet-pack mandarin sections (without liquid)
½ cup heavy-syrup mandarin sections
1 medium mango
1 large nectarine
1 large orange
1 medium papaya
2 medium peaches
¾ cup diet-pack peaches (without liquid)
½ cup heavy-syrup peaches
1 medium pear
¾ cup diet-pack pears (without liquid)
½ cup heavy-syrup pears
3 medium slices pineapple
½ cup chunk or crushed pineapple
¾ cup chunk diet-pack pineapple (without liquid)
3 medium plums
¾ cup diet-pack plums (without liquid)
½ cup heavy-syrup plums
½ pomegranate
½ cup diet-pack prunes (without liquid)
3 tablespoons dried raisins
1 cup black raspberries
1 cup red raspberries
5 cups fresh rhubarb
2 cups frozen unsweetened rhubarb
2 cups strawberries
2 cups frozen unsweetened strawberries
1 tangelo
2 large tangerines

2 Weight Watchers Fruit Snack or Apple Snack ½ oz.
   package, any flavor
2½ cups watermelon
1 entire 4½-oz. or 4¾-oz. jar of Gerber's applesauce,
   peaches, pears, apricots, plums, or pears and pineapple
1 entire 4½ oz. jar of Beechnut prunes with tapioca, or
   plums, pears, peaches, applesauce, or apricots with
   tapioca, or bananas and pineapple with tapioca, or apples
   and apricots, or bananas with tapioca (Baby foods are
   delicious toppings for cottage cheese, ice cream, muffins,
   etc.)

THE FRUIT JUICE STAND

6 oz. apple juice
6 oz. apricot nectar
6 oz. cranberry juice
16 oz. Ocean spray Low Calorie cranberry juice
8 oz. unsweetened grapefruit juice
8 oz. lemonade prepared from frozen concentrate or mix
6 oz. orange juice
6 oz. peach nectar
6 oz. pineapple juice
4 oz. prune juice
6 oz. Tang
6 oz. tangerine juice
16 oz. tomato juice
16 oz. vegetable juice cocktail

THE DRIED BEAN SACK

½ cup cooked and drained common white beans
½ cup cooked and drained cowpeas, immature or mature
½ cup cooked and drained lentils

½ cup cooked and drained lima beans, including frozen
½ cup cooked and drained pinto beans
½ cup cooked and drained red or kidney beans
½ cup cooked and drained green peas, immature
½ cup cooked and drained split peas, mature
½ cup cooked and drained soybeans, immature

The Butcher Block & The Fisherman's Net

Follow these instructions for enjoying The Butcher Block & The Fisherman's Net. (Where there is no brand name for an item, it is always *any brand*.) There are numerous groups from which you may select your one choice for the day and several ways you can treat this choice.

A. You may pick *one* choice
    or
B. You may pick *two* choices and simply divide the amount of each choice in *half*.

THE BUTCHER BLOCK

Important note: When selecting your meat, it is of the utmost importance that it be extremely *lean*. Just to give you an example about the different caloric values between the same cut of meat: According to the USDA, a 3½-oz. serving of cooked *lean* and *fat* club steak will yield 454 calories, whereas a 3½-oz. serving of *lean only* club steak will yield 244 calories. There is a tremendous difference of 210 calories just by selecting the lean cut. If you eat fatty cuts of meat or do not trim all visible fat you will increase your caloric intake with "wasted" calories. The leaner your meat, the better it is for you.

All choices are *lean only*, cooked trimmed of all visible fat, and ready to eat. Cooking method may be *any* providing that no additional fats are used and that juices rendered in the cooking process are not consumed.

4 oz. beef (suggested cuts: flank steak, round, london broil, foreshank, hindshank, chuck)

4 oz. lamb (suggested cuts: leg, shoulder)

4 oz. pork (suggested cuts: ham, picnic, boneless roast)

5 oz. chicken or turkey liver, or 4 oz. beef liver

4 oz. veal

4 oz. canned Oscar Mayer Jubilee boneless ham

10 slices or entire 6-oz. slice package of Oscar Mayer Smoked Cooked ham (95% fat-free)

4 oz. any commercially cured ham, very lean

1½ frankfurters packaged 10 to a pound, beef or with pork or fillers

2 of any brand chicken or turkey franks

8 Oscar Mayer Little Wieners

4 oz. Louis Rich Turkey Breakfast sausage

2½ oz. kielbasa

4 oz. duck, without skin

2½ oz. cooked soft salami

4 1-oz. slices Louis Rich turkey salami

4 oz. kidney, any kind

6 oz. venison

6 oz. dark or light meat turkey, without skin, or 4 oz. with
skin

6 oz. dark or light meat chicken, without skin, or 4 oz. with
skin

1 5-oz. can of Swanson Boned Turkey with Broth

1 5-oz. can of Swanson Chunk White Chicken with Broth

8 oz. plain tripe, including pickled or 3 oz. canned

5 medium slices bacon, cooked and well drained

3 oz. Canadian bacon, cooked and well drained

1 7-oz. container of Mrs. Kornberg's Chicken Liver (frozen)
chopped

3 links of Morning-Star Farms Cholesterol Free Breakfast
Links from the 8-oz. package, 10 links per packet

THE FISHERMAN'S NET

All choices are for cooked fish, ready to eat. The fish may
be prepared in any manner providing that no additional fats
are used in the cooking process. The cooked weight is without bones.

9 oz. abalone

6 oz. bass

5 oz. bluefish

6 oz. carp

5 oz. cod

8 oz. crappie

8 oz. crayfish

16 medium raw clams—all kinds

3 oz. frozen breaded and fried clams (to be baked only)
2 cups canned chopped or minced clams with liquid
2 6-oz. cartons of Wakefield Alaska King Crabmeat or with Shrimp (This is a fabulous selection!)
2 4-oz. jars of Sau-Sea Shrimp Cocktail
8 packaged frozen fish sticks (to be baked only)
8 oz. finnan haddie (also known as smoked haddock)
8 oz. flounder
12 oz. any kind of gefilte fish
10 oz. haddock
8 oz. Halibut, other than smoked
4 oz. pickled herring in brine
4 oz. kippered smoked herring
5 oz. herring in tomato sauce
10 oz. lobster
4 oz. smoked lox or Nova Scotia salmon, well drained
2 fish cakes from 8-oz. package, Mrs. Paul's (omit sauce)
Half of 7-oz. package of Mrs. Paul's French Fried Scallops (omit sauce)
Half of 7-oz. package of Mrs. Paul's Light Batter Scallops (omit sauce)
2 fried fish fillets from 8-oz. package, Mrs. Paul's
4 oz. mackerel other than salted or smoked
8 oz. mussels, meat only
1½ lb. mussels in shell
6 oz. ocean perch
12 oz. octopus
12 oz. oysters, meat only, or 24 medium oysters
8 oz. pike
8 oz. porgy
8 oz. red or gray snapper
8 oz. pink humpback fresh salmon steak
6 oz. canned salmon, any kind other than Atlantic
8 oz. scallops

4 oz. frozen breaded and fried scallops (to be baked only)

6 oz. shad

8 oz. shrimp

4 oz. frozen breaded and fried shrimp (to be baked only)

8 oz. smelt

8 oz. sole

10 oz. squid

6 oz. sturgeon, including smoked

8 oz. brook trout

4 oz. rainbow trout

5 oz. tuna, oil packed, very well drained

7 oz. tuna, water packed

3½ to 3¾ oz. can sardines, oil packed, very well drained

5 oz. sardines packed in mustard sauce or water

5 oz. sardines packed in tomato sauce

5½ oz. carton Mrs. Paul's Shrimp Crepes with Sauce

6 oz. whitefish

1½ 6-oz. packages of Gorton's Cod in Butter Sauce *or*

1½ 6-oz. packages of Gorton's Cod in Cheese Sauce

Although the following are not in the meat or fish family, you may use them as substitutes for variety.

OTHER PROTEIN SOURCES

2½ tablespoons peanut butter

3 large eggs

12 oz. 99% fat-free cottage cheese

2½ oz. hard cheese other than sweet dessert type

7 oz. soybeans, mature seed, cooked and drained

12 oz. tofu (soybean curd)

1 8-oz. package Weight Watchers Imitation Cream Cheese

The Soup Tureen & The Juice Pitcher

Follow these instructions for enjoying The Soup Tureen & The Juice Pitcher. (Where there is no brand name for an item, it is always *any brand*.)

You may pick *one* choice.

THE SOUP TUREEN

Important note: All choices represent a 6-oz. serving that has been prepared according to package directions using *water* only, or as otherwise noted.

Campbell's

Chicken Gumbo
Chicken Noodle
Chicken with Rice
Onion
Old Fashioned Vegetable
Chicken broth
Consomme
Turkey vegetable
Chicken & Stars

Crosse & Blackwell

1 13-oz. can Clear Consommé Madrilene

Doxsee

Manhattan Clam Chowder

Lipton

1 packet Beef n' Noodles Cup-a-Soup
1 packet Chicken Noodle Cup-a-Soup
1 packet Spring Vegetable Cup-a-Soup
Chicken Noodle with Diced White Chicken Meat
Onion
Vegetable Beef
Alphabet Vegetable

Manischewitz

Beef Cabbage
Tomato
Vegetarian Vegetable
5 cups Schav
Borscht, plain
16 oz. low-calorie Borscht

Progresso

1 entire can (19½-oz.) Escarole in Chicken Broth. (Yes!
Enjoy it all—delicious hot or cold!)

THE JUICE PITCHER

8 oz. tomato juice
8 oz. vegetable juice cocktail
4 oz. orange juice

4 oz. grapefruit juice
8 oz. low-calorie Ocean spray cranberry juice
1½ cups Doxsee or Snow's Clam Juice

The Hen's Nest, The Cheese Shed & The Deli

Follow these instructions for enjoying The Hen's Nest, The Cheese Shed & The Deli. (Where there is no brand name for an item, it is always *any brand*). There are numerous groups from which you may select your one choice for the day and several ways you can treat this choice.

A. You may pick *one* choice
   or
B. You may pick *two* choices and simply divide the amount of each choice in *half*.

THE HEN'S NEST

2 small eggs, brown or white
1 extra large or jumbo egg, brown or white
7 egg whites—marvelous when hard-boiled. Use for filling and making low-calorie, high-protein delicious egg boats that can be stuffed with a variety of fillings.
¾ cup Fleischmann's egg beaters

THE CHEESE SHED

6 oz. 99% fat-free cottage cheese, unflavored (¾ cup)

4 oz. regular cottage cheese, unflavored (½ cup)

3 oz. farmer cheese

3 tablespoons plain whipped cream cheese

3 tablespoons grated Cheddar cheese

3 tablespoons grated Parmesan or Romano cheese

1 oz. any kind of cheese other than sweet dessert type

2 oz. low-fat skimmed milk or regular ricotta

2 slices of Lite-line pasteurized process cheese from the 12 single-wrap slice pack

7 The Laughing Cow (la vache qui rit) Cheezbits, from the 4-oz. package

3 wedges reduced calories The Laughing Cow (la vache qui rit) green label

2 ⅓-oz. servings Weight Watchers Imitation Cream Cheese

THE DELI

2 slices bacon, cooked and drained

1 oz. bologna

1 oz. braunschweiger liver sausage or liverwurst

2 oz. Underwood Chunky Chicken Spread

2 oz. Underwood Corned Beef Spread

2 tablespoons Sell's canned Liver Pate

3 oz. ham, lean

5 slices Oscar Mayer Smoked Cooked Ham (95% fat-free)

3½ oz. tuna, canned in *water*

2 oz. turkey roll

2 oz. chicken roll

1 Longacre chicken frank

1 Weaver chicken frank

4 Oscar Mayer Little Wieners
1 tablespoon peanut butter
5 slices Louis Rich Smoked Turkey Breast
2 slices Louis Rich Turkey Bologna
3 slices Louis Rich Turkey Pastrami
1 Louis Rich Turkey frank
¾ oz. soy nuts

The Tiny Items That Make A Big Sensation & The Pub

Follow these instructions for enjoying The Tiny Items That Make a Big Sensation & The Pub. There are numerous groups from which you may select your two choices for the day and several ways you can treat these choices.

A. You may pick the same choice *twice*
   or
B. You may pick *two* different choices
   or
C. You may pick *four* different choices and divide the amount of each choice in *half*.

Caution: Some items represent 2 choices. Example: The Chocolate Factory, The Candy Store, The Nutcracker. Read carefully!

THE TINY ITEMS THAT MAKE A BIG SENSATION

THE GRAVY BOAT

2 tablespoons cornstarch

2 tablespoons all-purpose flour

¼ cup gravy mix that has been prepared according to package directions. French's, Durkee, Pillsbury or McCormick, any variety (omit gravy drippings in preparation)

1 entire 10½ oz. can of Franco-American Au Jus Gravy

1 entire box (⅝ oz.) Pillsbury's Gravy Mix, Brown or Home-Style

1 packet any variety gravy surprise Weight Watchers gravy mix

1 entire 0.5-oz. (14.1 grams) package Weight Watchers Chicken Gravy Mix

1 entire 0.44-oz. (12.4 grams) package Weight Watchers Brown Gravy Mix

THE CREAM PITCHER

3 tablespoons half and half

4 tablespoons Perx

2 tablespoons Pream

1 tablespoon heavy whipping cream

4 teaspoons Cremora

THE SUGAR AND HONEY BOWL

2 tablespoons sifted confectioners' sugar

1 tablespoon brown or white sugar

1 tablespoon honey

THE CONDIMENT JAR

4 tablespoons any kind relish
3 tablespoons ketchup
4 tablespoons chili sauce
3 tablespoons cocktail sauce
5 tablespoons barbecue sauce
1 tablespoon tartar sauce

THE SPRINKLE SHAKER

3 tablespoons fresh shredded coconut
¼ cup Durkee shredded coconut
4 tablespoons imitation bacon bits
3 tablespoons bread crumbs
2 tablespoons any kind grated cheese
5 tablespoons dehydrated onion flakes

THE OLD FASHIONED JAMS & JELLIES

2 tablespoons apple butter
4 teaspoons any variety jam or jelly
9 teaspoons Smucker's Low Sugar Spread, any flavor
1 tablespoon honey

TO TOP IT OFF

4 tablespoons any type whipped topping such as Cool
    Whip, etc.
2 tablespoons sour cream
2 tablespoons caviar

PLEASE PASS THE SYRUP

2 tablespoons Hershey's chocolate syrup
1 tablespoon maple-flavored syrup
5 tablespoons Diet Delight Pancake and Waffle Topping
Unlimited use of Cary's artificial Maple Low-Calorie Syrup
  (no calories!)
10 teaspoons Diet Delight or Tillie Lewis pancake and
  waffle syrup

THE CHOCOLATE FACTORY

Note: (Each item represents *two* choices)

1 package of M & M's Plain Chocolate Candies from the
  7⅞-oz. box, or about 22 pieces
1 1.05-oz. Hershey's Milk Chocolate
1 1.2-oz. package of Reese's Milk Chocolate (2 Peanut
  Butter Cups)
4 Hershey's Assorted Miniatures from the 6-oz. package
16 Estee Dietetic Chocolate TV Mix individual candies
1 1⅛-oz. KitKat crisp wafers in chocolate
6 Hershey's Kisses

THE CANDY STORE

Note: (Each item represents two choices)

16 Life Savers, any flavor
80 Kraft or Campfire Miniature Marshmallows
6 pieces of Pearson Coffee Nip
12 Nabisco Chuckles Ju jubes
1 ¾-oz. bar of Sahadi Sesame Crunch

THE BRAND NAME DIET

THE GUM BALL MACHINE

6 sticks any flavor gum
15 pieces Dentyne
10 Chicklets, any flavor
10 sticks dietetic gum, any flavor

THE ICE-CREAM TRUCK

1 2½-fl. oz. Welch's Grape Bar
1 Good Humor Fruit Stix, any flavor, 1.5 fl. oz.
1 plain vanilla Danny yogurt on a stick
3 plain (not rolled sugar) ice-cream cones, cone *only*
1 rolled sugar ice-cream cone, cone *only*
1 Popsicle, all flavors, except chocolate
1 3-oz. cup Carvel Thinny Thin, any flavor
1 small chocolate Dairy Queen Sundae (this represents *two*
   choices)

LET'S GO TO THE MOVIES

3 cups any kind popped corn without added butter, plain
1 bag of any selection from Frito-Lay variety pack (this
   includes corn chips, nacho cheese flavored tortilla chips,
   and potato chips)
½-oz. package of Wise potato chips from the snack pack
   containing 8 packages
70 Nabisco mister salty Veri-Thin Pretzel Sticks

THE NUT CRACKER

Note: (Each item represents *two* choices)

1 oz. shelled almonds
1 oz. shelled butternuts

1 oz. dry-roasted cashews
2 oz. fresh, shelled chestnuts
1 oz. Planters dry-roasted mixed nuts
1 oz. Planters dry-roasted peanuts
2 oz. pistachios, in shell
1 oz. soybean nuts

THE SEED BAG

(Note: Each item represents *two* choices)

1 oz. hulled pumpkin seeds
1 oz. hulled sesame seeds
2 oz. sunflower seeds in hulls
1 oz. hulled, dry-roasted sunflower seeds

THE INCREDIBLE SPREADABLES

5 teaspoons any variety Nabisco Snackmate canned cheese
spread
3 tablespoons anchovy paste
2 tablespoons Underwood Corned Beef Spread
1 tablespoon any sandwich spread
2 tablespoons Sell's canned Liver Pate

THE HORS D'OEUVRES TRAY

1 oz. caviar, black or red
2 Chun King cocktail-size shrimp egg rolls, ½-oz. size
2 Chun King cocktail-size chicken egg rolls, ½-oz. size
2 Chun King cocktail-size lobster and meat egg rolls, ½-oz.
size
2 Jenos pizza rolls, any variety
2 Patio cocktail size beef tacos, ½-oz. size

POTPOURRI

5 egg whites (hard-boiled for filling; raw for whipping)
4 lemons or limes
1 Lawry's taco or tostada shell
12 medium green or black olives
2 teaspoons Nestlé's Quik
4 oz. soybean curd (tofu)
8 cough drops, any variety
4 maraschino cherries, any brand
1 (0.56 oz.) package Lawry's Green Onion or Toasted Onion
    Dip Mix

THE PUB

THE KEG OF BEER

6 oz. beer
8 oz. beer that is 100 calories or less per 12 oz.

THE LIQUOR CASE

1 oz. unflavored bourbon whiskey, brandy, Canadian
    whiskey, gin, Irish whiskey, rum, rye whiskey, Scotch
    whiskey, Tequila or vodka

THE WINE CELLAR

3 oz. very dry red or white wine

THE CORDIAL DECANTER

¾ oz. any cordial or liqueur

THE CHAMPAGNE BUCKET

3 oz. champagne

THE PARTY MIXER

1 envelope (1 serving) of any dry cocktail mix

The Salad Bowl

Here are delightful crunchy fixings for your salads. When used *raw*, they may be mixed and matched in *any* amount. There is no limit as to how much or how often you may treat yourself to The Salad Bowl.

cauliflower	parsley
celery	green peppers
chicory	red peppers
chives	pimentos
endive	radishes
escarole	scallions
lettuce	spinach
mushrooms	watercress

The Salad Dressing, Butter & Bacon Corner

Follow these instructions for enjoying The Salad Dressing, Butter & Bacon Corner. (Where there is no brand name for an item, it is always *any brand*.) There are numerous groups from which you may select your one choice for the day and several ways you can treat this choice.

A. You may pick *one* choice
   or
B. You may pick *two* choices and simply divide the amount of each choice in *half*.

THE SALAD DRESSING

Important note: All salad dressings are 2 tablespoons unless otherwise specified.

Kraft

Roka Blue Cheese
Russian
Casino
Thousand Island

Lawry's

Blue or Bleu Cheese
California, French
San Francisco, Garlic
Green Goddess
Italian with Cheese
Sherry

Wish-Bone

deluxe French
Russian

LOW-CALORIE AND LIGHT SALAD DRESSINGS—BOTTLED

Any type or brand up to 120 calories represents *one* choice.

THE BUTTER AND BACON CORNER

12 teaspoons imitation bacon bits
3 medium slices bacon, very well drained
3½ teaspoons butter
5 teaspoons whipped butter
3½ teaspoons margarine
7 teaspoons imitation diet margarine
1 tablespoon any kind of oil
1 tablespoon real mayonnaise
2 tablespoons Kraft imitation mayonnaise
5 teaspoons Kraft Miracle Whip
4 tablespoons sour cream
2 individual ½-oz. foil packets from the 4-oz. box of Butter
   Buds

To Your Heart's Content

You may have as much as desired from the following.

THE HERB GARDEN

basil, bay leaves, dill, marjoram, mint, oregano, parsley, rosemary, sage, tarragon, thyme, etc.

THE SPICE RACK

chili powder, cinnamon, cloves, cumin, curry, ginger, nutmeg, paprika, pepper, allspice, saffron, etc.

THE CONDIMENT & SEASONING JAR

Accent, horseradish (white or red), garlic salt, mustard, MSG (monosodium glutamate), onion salt, vinegar, soy sauce, salt, seasoned salt, tabasco, Worcestershire sauce, etc.

THE FLAVORINGS

all flavored extracts, all flavors No-Cal syrups

THE DESSERT DISH

all flavors dietetic gelatin, rennet tablets

THE SODA FOUNTAIN

all dietetic carbonated beverages (soda and soft drinks)

THE WATER COOLER

club soda, mineral water, seltzer, spring water, water

THE COFFEE URN

all imported and domestic varieties of instant, decaffeinated or ground coffees

THE TEAPOT

all imported and domestic varieties of teas. These may be flavored, such as mint, peppermint, jasmine, etc.

THE BROTH MUG

all flavors of broth from cubes or packets

THE SUGAR BOWL

any type of artificial sweetner

THE SPRAY N' FRY PAN

any brand of spray-on pan coating

The International Buffet

Important note: When choosing from The International Buffet, on that day, just skip the following categories:

③ The Vegetable Patch, The Fruit Stand & The Dried Bean Sack
   and
④ The Butcher Block & The Fisherman's Net
   and
⑤ The Soup Tureen & The Juice Pitcher
For nutritional balance, go to ⑧ The Salad Bowl.

Follow these instructions for enjoying The International Buffet. There are numerous groups from which you may select your one choice for the day and several ways you can treat this choice.

A. You may pick *one* choice each day
   or
B. You may pick *two* choices and divide the amount of each choice in *half.*

THE U.S.A.

1 11-oz. frozen fried chicken dinner, Morton
1 entire 15-oz. can of Swanson's beef stew

1 16-oz. dinner of Weight Watchers Sliced Breast of Turkey

1 6½-oz. package of Stouffer's Creamed Chicken

2 frozen 9-oz. Boil 'n Bags, Chicken & Noodles, Green Giant

1 8-oz. frozen beef pie, Banquet, Swanson or Morton

1 8-oz. frozen chicken pie, Banquet, Swanson or Morton

1 8-oz. frozen turkey pie, Banquet, Swanson, or Morton

2 7-oz. entree servings of Green Giant Frozen Stuffed Cabbage

1 10½-oz. frozen Weight Watchers Chicken Livers and Onions

ITALY

10 Jenos pizza rolls, any variety—12 to a package

1 15-oz. can Chef Boy-ar-dee Ravioli in sauce

1 15-oz. can Franco-American Beef Ravioli with meat sauce

1 14¾-oz. can Franco-American Spaghetti-O's with little meatballs

2 13-oz. packages of Weight Watchers Eggplant Parmigiana

2 frozen 9-oz. Weight Watchers Chicken Parmigiana with Spinach

1 13-oz. package Weight Watchers Lasagna with Cheese, Veal and Sauce

1 13-oz. package Weight Watchers Veal Stuffed Pepper in Sauce

1 13-oz. package Weight Watchers Turkey Tetrazzini Au Gratin

1 13-oz. package Weight Watchers Ziti Macaroni with Veal, Cheese and Sauce

1 7½-oz. package Gorton's Shrimp Scampi

2 8-oz. frozen Ronzoni Baked Ziti complete with sauce

2 8-oz. Frozen Ronzoni Single Serving Macaroni & Eggplant Casserole

THE BRAND NAME DIET

1 8-oz. frozen Ronzoni Fettucine Alfredo
1 7-oz. frozen Celeste cheese pizza
1 7-oz. frozen Weight Watchers sausage pizza

CHINA

4 9-oz. entrees of frozen Green Giant Chicken Chow Mein
1 16-oz. carton La Choy Shrimp Chow Mein, frozen
1 16-oz. carton La Choy Chicken Chow Mein, frozen
1 6½-oz. carton La Choy Egg Rolls, frozen (15 per box)
1 6½-oz. carton La Choy Lobster Egg Rolls, frozen (15 per box)
5 cups frozen La Choy Won Ton Soup
3 16-oz. cans La Choy beef, chicken, or shrimp chow mein
3 16-oz. cans La Choy Fancy Mixed Chinese Vegetables
1½ 16-oz. can Chun King beef, chicken or shrimp chow mein
1½ cups any brand chow mein noodles
1 8- or 8½-oz. can any brand water chestnuts
1 11-oz. can La Choy fried rice

MEXICO

1¼ cups chili con carne, with or without beans, any brand
1 13-oz. dinner of beef enchilada, Patio
1 12-oz. dinner of cheese enchilada, Patio or Banquet
1½ cups refried beans, any brand
8 taco shells, any brand
1 7½-oz. can Old El Paso Beef Taco Filling
4 canned Beef Tamales, any brand
2 6-oz. frozen bags Banquet beef enchiladas
12 ½-oz. cocktail tacos, Patio
1½ 11-oz. cans of Campbell's Chunky Soup, Chili Beef

FRANCE

2 5½-oz. frozen packages Mrs. Paul's crepes—any variety
1 8-oz. frozen package Mrs. Paul's Fillet of Sole, Breaded &
 Fried
1 9-oz. frozen package of Gorton's Fillet of Sole in Lemon
 Butter
10 Durkee beef or shrimp puffs
5 oz. Sell's or Hormel liver pâté
4 frozen slices of Aunt Jemima French Toast from 9-oz. box

How to Eat at McDonald's, Burger King, Etc.

(The Great Getaway to the Land of Fast Foods)

This category allows you to eat out with your family and friends without having to sit and stare and nurse a glass of water!

What follows are numerous **Trade-Offs.** If, for instance, you would like to enjoy a hamburger from McDonald's you will have to trade it off for the one choice to which you are entitled in The Butcher Block & The Fisherman's Net. Or if you would like to delight in a small chocolate sundae from Dairy Queen you will have to trade it off for the two choices to which you are entitled from The Tiny Items That Make a Big Sensation & The Pub.

McDONALD'S

1 Egg McMuffin = skip The Hen's Nest, The Cheese Shed
& The Deli; The Bakery, Cereal Bowl & Grain Bin and
The Salad Dressing, Butter & Bacon Corner

1 portion scrambled eggs = skip The Hen's Nest, The
Cheese Shed & The Deli and The Soup Tureen & The
Juice Pitcher

1 hamburger = skip The Butcher Block & The Fisherman's
Net

1 cheeseburger = skip The Butcher Block & The
Fisherman's Net and The Soup Tureen & The Juice
Pitcher

1 small french fries = skip 2 choices The Vegetable Patch,
The Fruit Stand & The Dried Bean Sack

1 regular vanilla shake = skip The Milk Barn & The Ice
Cream Parlor; The Tiny Items That Make a Big Sensation
& The Pub and the Soup Tureen & The Juice Pitcher

1 strawberry or pineapple sundae = skip The Milk Barn &
The Ice-Cream Parlor and The Hen's Nest, The Cheese
Shed & The Deli

DAIRY QUEEN

1 Single Burger = skip The Butcher Block & The
Fisherman's Net and The Salad Dressing, Butter & Bacon
Corner

The Brazier Dog = skip The Butcher Block & The
Fisherman's Net

The Brazier Cheese Dog = skip The Butcher Block & The
Fisherman's Net and The Hen's Nest, The Cheese Shed
& The Deli

french fries (small—2.5-oz.) = skip The Vegetable Patch,
The Fruit Stand & The Dried Bean Sack

chocolate dipped cone, small = skip The Tiny Items That Make a Big Sensation & The Pub

chocolate sundae, small = skip The Tiny Items That Make a Big Sensation & The Pub

onion rings = skip The Vegetable Patch, The Fruit Stand & The Dried Bean Sack and The Salad Dressing, Butter & Bacon Corner

The Fish Sandwich = skip The Butcher Block & The Fisherman's Net and The Bakery, Cereal Bowl & Grain Bin

1 small plain cone = skip The Milk Barn & The Ice-Cream Parlor

JACK IN THE BOX

1 Regular Taco = skip The Vegetable Patch, The Fruit Stand & The Dried Bean Sack

1 Super Taco = skip The Butcher Block & The Fisherman's Net and The Soup Tureen & The Juice Pitcher

1 Breakfast Jack = skip The Butcher Block & The Fisherman's Net and The Soup Tureen & The Juice Pitcher

1 hamburger = skip The Butcher Block & The Fisherman's Net

1 Cheeseburger = skip The Butcher Block & The Fisherman's Net and The Soup Tureen & The Juice Pitcher

1 vanilla shake = skip The Tiny Items That Make a Big Sensation & The Pub and The Soup Tureen & The Juice Pitcher and The Milk Barn & The Ice Cream Parlor

BURGER KING

1 hamburger = skip The Butcher Block & The Fisherman's Net and The Soup Tureen & The Juice Pitcher

1 hamburger with cheese = skip The Butcher Block & The

Fisherman's Net and The Hen's Nest, The Cheese Shed
& The Deli

1 regular french fries = skip two choices in The Vegetable
Patch, The Fruit Stand & The Dried Bean Sack

1 chocolate or vanilla shake = skip The Milk Barn & The
Ice-Cream Parlor; The Tiny Items That Make a Big
Sensation & The Pub and The Soup Tureen & The Juice
Pitcher

1 apple pie = skip The Tiny Items That Make a Big
Sensation & The Pub and The Salad Dressing, Butter &
Bacon Corner

1 small onion rings = skip The Tiny Items That Make a Big
Sensation & The Pub and The Salad Dressing, Butter &
Bacon Corner

ARTHUR TREACHER'S

1 chowder = skip The Hen's Nest, The Cheese Shed & The
Deli

2 pieces fish = skip The Butcher Block & The Fisherman's
Net and The Salad Dressing, Butter & Bacon Corner

1 Fish Sandwich = skip The Butcher Block & The
Fisherman's Net; The Tiny Items That Make a Big
Sensation & The Pub and The Soup Tureen & The Juice
Pitcher

1 Chicken Sandwich = skip The Butcher Block & The
Fisherman's Net; The Tiny Items That Make a Big
Sensation & The Pub and The Soup Tureen & The Juice
Pitcher

1 cole slaw = skip The Salad Dressing, Butter & Bacon
Corner

7 pieces shrimp = skip The Butcher Block & The
Fisherman's Net and The Salad Dressing, Butter & Bacon
Corner

PIZZA HUT

2 slices medium Thin n' Crispy, standard cheese = skip
   The Bakery, Cereal Bowl & Grain Bin; The Hen's Nest,
   The Cheese Shed & The Deli and The Soup Tureen & The
   Juice Pitcher
2 slices medium Thin n' Crispy, standard pepperoni = skip
   The Bakery, Cereal Bowl & Grain Bin; The Hen's Nest,
   The Cheese Shed & The Deli and The Salad Dressing,
   Butter & Bacon Corner

KENTUCKY FRIED CHICKEN

(original recipe)
2 drumsticks = skip The Butcher Block & The Fisherman's
   Net
1 thigh = skip The Butcher Block & The Fisherman's Net
1 keel = skip The Butcher Block & The Fisherman's Net
1 rib = skip The Butcher Block & The Fisherman's Net and
   The Soup Tureen & The Juice Pitcher
1 mashed potato with gravy = skip The Salad Dressing,
   Butter & Bacon Corner
1 cole slaw = skip The Salad Dressing, Butter & Bacon
   Corner
1 potato salad = skip The Salad Dressing, Butter & Bacon
   Corner
1 Kentucky crisp fries, small = skip The Bakery, Cereal
   Bowl & Grain Bin

V

Calorie Counts of The
Brand Name Diet

In order to demystify the diet for you, I have given approximate calorie values below for each of the twelve categories. Note that there can be a 10- to 20- and even sometimes a 50-calorie differential between all choices in any one given category. However, the differential above the limit is no more than 30 calories. The 50-calorie differential is always below the limit. You need not worry about which selection is higher or lower in calories. The diet is designed to balance itself out predicated on the fact that you will balance out the choices.

The approximate calorie counts are as follows:

① The Bakery, Cereal Bowl & Grain Bin: **160**
② The Milk Barn & The Ice-Cream Parlor: **120**
③ The Vegetable Patch, The Fruit Stand & The Dried Bean Sack: **200**

④ The Butcher Block & The Fisherman's Net: **250**
⑤ The Soup Tureen & The Juice Pitcher: **50**
⑥ The Hen's Nest, The Cheese Shed & The Deli: **120**
⑦ The Tiny Items That Make a Big Sensation & The Pub: **160**
⑧ The Salad Bowl: **50**
⑨ The Salad Dressing, Butter & Bacon Corner: **120**
⑩ To Your Heart's Content: **50**

The International Buffet and How to Eat at McDonald's, Etc. are a combination of many categories; therefore it is not feasible to give you specific calorie counts. Figuring the calorie counts yourself will become easier for you the more you read the preceding chapter, the diet itself.

You have been given the calorie counts so that should you encounter a food which I have not listed, you have the ability to then incorporate it into one of the categories. You may find that you are looking for many items which do not appear. Clearly, it was virtually impossible to please all tastes. I have tried my best to reach a broad audience of dieters, but since I believe that individuality is one of the most important aspects of dieting, you can now put your own signature to your own version of *The Brand Name Diet* by inserting your own goodies. And that is part of the magic!

You can consult calorie counter books, such as *Calories and Carbohydrates*, by Barbara Kraus, to find out how many calories there are in foods you'd like to incorporate in your Brand Name Diet. Just how much flexibility you have with this diet depends on you. It is not my intention to have the last word and shout absolutes at you. Quite the contrary: Freedom and independence for you are an integral part of the success of *The Brand Name Diet*.

VI

Fascinating Finds and Comparisons

As we come to the close of the nutritional section of *The Brand Name Diet*, I want to remind you that comparing foods and being very careful about selecting your choices on sight at the supermarket is mandatory for your weight loss. I have included some incredible little finds which I would like to share with you:

1 pound raw beef flank steak yields 653 calories, whereas 1 pound raw beef club steak (boneless) yields 1,724 calories!

One cup of Del Monte yellow cling sliced peaches in heavy syrup yields 170 calories, whereas one cup of Libby's Lite sliced yellow cling peaches in real fruit juice yields 100 calories. In this instance, you are not getting any more bulk for your calories; to the contrary, you are getting unnecessary sugars and corn sweeteners.

You can have twice as much natural-style Mott's Apple Sauce without sugar or preservatives added as you can for their same brand containing sugar and corn sweetener. What a bonus to the dieter!—Better nutrition for fewer calories.

1 Danny uncoated vanilla frozen lowfat yogurt on a stick has only 60 calories, whereas 1 carob boysenberry Danny frozen yogurt on a stick has 140 calories!

Brady's markets unsweetened frozen fruits which count the same as a portion of fresh fruit.

You might ask yourself why it is that I have included two packets of Alba 66 for 120 calories and have not included two packets of Ovaltine Reduced Calorie Cocoa Mix yielding 100 calories. The reason is the Ovaltine choice gives you only 2 grams of protein whereas the Alba choice gives you a bonus of 12 grams of protein.

One large whole egg contains 80 calories and 7 grams of protein, whereas you can now get egg beaters, cholesterol-free egg substitute from Fleischmann's, at half a cup for 80 calories. This half-cup is equivalent to 2 eggs and 14 grams protein. In other words, you can eat double the amount of egg beaters for the same calorie and protein investment of one large egg.

In this comparison of four delicious frozen confections, ½ cup (4 oz.) of vanilla yields significantly different amounts of calories, fat, carbohydrates, and protein.

Häagen Dazs Ice Cream
267 calories
  16 grams fat

25 grams carbohydrates
5 grams protein

Light n' Lively Ice Milk
100 calories
2 grams fat
17 grams carbohydrates
3 grams protein

Breyers Ice Cream
140 calories
8 grams fat
15 grams carbohydrates
3 grams protein

Sealtest Ice Cream
140 calories
7 grams fat
16 grams carbohydrates
2 grams protein

4 yeast raised plain Dunkin' Donuts Munchkins total only 104 calories, whereas 1 Dunkin' Donuts Cruller yields 240 calories!

6 fluid ounces of regular Ocean spray Cranberry Juice Cocktail yields 110 calories, whereas 6 ounces of their low-calorie juice has only 35!

2 teaspoons of Smucker's strawberry jelly yields 35 calories, whereas 2 teaspoons of Smucker's Low Calorie Strawberry Spread yields 16 calories.

New to the supermarket are a series of low-fat fruited yogurt products. Read their labels very carefully. For instance: An 8-ounce container of Dannon strawberry yogurt contains 260 calories, whereas an 8-ounce container of Sweet n' Low strawberry nonfat yogurt contains 150 calories.

One 9-ounce portion of Gorton's Fillet of Sole seafood entree contains 400 calories whereas one 6-ounce package of Gorton's Cod in Butter Sauce yields 170 calories.

Diet Delight packs 2 kinds of fruits. Those with the green label are packed in water with no sugar added. Those with the blue label are packed in juice from concentrate of white grapes. Let's look at a calorie comparison. Half a cup under the blue label of unpeeled halved apricots yields 60 calories, whereas half a cup under the green label of unpeeled halved apricots yields 35 calories. Simply add your own no-calorie sweetener to the green can and you have saved yourself 25 calories!

One 8-ounce frozen Ronzoni Single Serving Baked Ziti complete with sauce yields 250 calories, whereas one 8-ounce package of Ronzoni Fettucine Alfredo yields an incredibly high 430 calories!

1 lb. whole raw Chinook or King salmon yields 886 calories, whereas 1 lb. whole raw pink or humpback salmon yields 475 calories!

There is more to dieting than diet. The nutritional and physical changes that will be occurring with your dieting efforts make up only one aspect of your quest for slimness. The next chapter will deal with the psychological aspects.

VII

Food Around Us

It would be very difficult or nearly impossible to live through one day without being subjected to food advertising in one form or another. In order to escape all this temptation we would have to enclose ourselves in a soundproof, lightproof, mediaproof environment. Let's look at what our eyes and ears are fed each day:

- Walking up and down the colorful **supermarket** aisles
- Listening to the ad about the wonderful home-baked taste of bread over the **radio**
- Looking at a pint of ice cream emerge from its container on **television**
- Thumbing through a **newspaper** and seeing the display ads for food stores
- Staring at a **billboard** picturing a jumbo cheeseburger, french fries and Coke
- Passing a delicatessen and seeing a **sign** about potato chips
- Reading a **magazine** and seeing those fabulous displays of cakes and cookies

The sole purpose of food advertising is to make food so appealing to us that we feel we must try it. The better the ad, the more people will buy the food, the more revenue the food company will make—the more trouble we get into!

We may not desire any particular food, but just *hearing* or *seeing* a suggestion of it starts our wheels turning. We can almost *taste* the maple syrup as it is slowly poured over a stack of steaming pancakes. It almost seems to ooze out of the screen. We don't need the syrup in order to survive, but the syrup company depends on our consuming it for their survival.

We can almost *smell* the aroma of the freshly baked bread from the radio. We can almost *visualize* ourselves frosting the latest cake recipe of the month, presented to us in those dazzling, spectacular, full-page magazine displays. Using frosting is not essential to our lives, but it *is* essential to the life of the frosting company.

The temptation is almost overwhelming to take advantage of the "last chance" of buying the candy and gum so invitingly displayed on racks beside supermarket checkout counters. And how about those nifty little coupons that we find in countless boxes of snacks, inviting us to save 7 cents on our next purchase!

Advertising does perhaps its most effective job on children. They are an innocent audience: children do not know the nutritive value and difference between cottage cheese and a cupcake. Children do not know that there is a company behind the cupcake, one that depends on the purchase of their products. These commercials are very carefully geared to a child's level. So children are taught to associate cookies, ice cream bars, sugary drinks, etc., with having fun, making friends, enjoying climbing a tree, going fishing or swimming. Snack food companies deftly zero in on unsuspecting kids. The commercials tell them that eating these foods is the "in" thing to do. Commercials can have such clout that sometimes when our children demand one product or another we buy it in order to still their requests. Or if we refrain from buying something, we feel "guilty" because in some distorted way we believe we may be depriving them.

Overweight people, on the other hand, are the prey of the diet food industry. Some so-called diet products have the same number of calories as a regularly packaged product. We can be misled by labels such as "Absolutely no sugar added. Only pure honey." For lack of knowledge, we may think that this means the food has fewer calories because it is in the diet section. Actually, honey is higher in caloric value, with a count of 61 calories per tablespoon in comparison to 46 calories for 1 tablespoon of granulated sugar. This is not to say that sugar is preferred to honey. Just be sure you've compared the quantities used and the resulting calorie count before assuming that a food has fewer calories. Do not be persuaded by ads. Look into each matter yourself and then decide!

In conclusion, whether it be the thrust of advertising, the arousal of one of the strong food senses or emotional pressure, check out with your own mind just why you are reaching for food. Is it real hunger or something else?

VIII

The Psychology Behind
The Brand Name Diet

DIETING GAMES AND HOW TO
STOP PLAYING THEM

Here I'm going to present some of the most common dieting games. Without playing games such as these, we would not be fat. All of these are defense mechanisms we use to protect ourselves from reality in order to give ourselves permission to binge. I am going to show you how the out-of-control part of your personality creates havoc in your life. For purposes of identification we will call the irrational part of your personality the *Alternate*.

You will witness what your Alternate is capable of doing to you and how you can take away its harmful effects, rendering it powerless so that you can take control in any given situation. You will be amazed to discover how your Alternate can strangle the life right out of all your dieting attempts!

THE BRAND NAME DIET

1. The Search For the Miracle Game.

How and why we play the game: We constantly search for an instant, painless and everlasting cure for our weight problem, and/or we cover our lack of self-confidence by giving ourselves up to some sensational power. It is very understandable that we are drawn to the latest wonder pill, the most recent inflatable sauna suit, the newest chewing gum appetite curber, the most fabulous weighted belt exerciser, the most fantastic combination of health food derivatives, and countless other wonders. Who wouldn't want to lose 7 pounds in just forty-eight hours by simply swallowing a capsule, and who wouldn't want to lose 5 inches off his or her waist and 10 pounds in seven days by wearing some kind of contraption three times a day?

How to stop playing the game: Recognize that the miracle is never brought in from the outside; it always lies within you. You can and will reach deep down into yourself to awaken your self-reliance. Dealing with reality is in itself a miracle.

2. The On-and-Off Scale-Hop Game.

How and why we play the game: We use the scale to see how much we have gotten away with in a binge. We kid ourselves by shifting the scale around to find where it gives the lowest weight possible. The scale becomes the only means of reward, the only motivation to keep going. We believe it is broken if it does not give us the answers we want.

How to stop playing the game: Use the scale sparingly as a means of judging the effectiveness of diet modifications, and as only *one* of the instruments of encouragement.

3. The "I'll Take a Few Diet Pills to Get Me Started" Game.

How and why we play the game: This game is sometimes played in order to attain an initial rapid weight loss without the use of any self-control, thinking that the weight loss will somehow continue of its own accord even when the pills are used up, or to ease the pain of reaching a plateau when we find outselves stuck. We reach for artificial help when we don't feel capable of trying harder.

How to stop playing the game: The diet pills are a means to a dead end in more ways than one.

1. They can be habit-forming, not only physically, but psychologically
2. They most often do the job they are expected to, namely, giving a weight loss only because the pill controls you

This kind of external control teaches us only one form of discipline—to take the pills on time. Once the pills are withdrawn, we find ourselves left with an emotional dependence on them. Most often we return to the diet pills, promising ourselves that they will be used only to get started just once more. Thus the vicious cycle is set in motion time after time after time. (It must be stated here that when anorexiants are used under close medical supervision for very specific cases, they do have a place in medical practice. However, these cases are few and far between.)

4. The "I'm Only Buying It For So-and-So" Game.

How and why we play the game: We sometimes buy goodies under the guise of needing them for someone else—to prepare for unexpected company, satisfy pressure from the kids ("I want this, I want that"), treat our spouses with that special dessert, or please Cousin Blanche who is coming next month and I had better buy her favorite cookies now lest they be out of stock when she's here.

How to stop playing the game: Whenever possible go to the supermarket on a full stomach. While pushing that cart up and down the aisles of boxes, jars, packages, bags, bottles and containers that seem to be saying "Buy me, buy me," be armed with food you can conveniently munch on right up to the cash register if necessary. You must recognize that the purchasing of food is the first step leading to all the eating games. If you shop judiciously and are aware of what you are doing, you have a head start on the road to modifying your behavior.

5. The "As Long As It's Diet Food, It's Okay" Game.

How and why we play the game: As long as we are doing something connected with the word "diet," we are in the process of trying to become slim and we must be doing something right. We make ourselves feel good as we purchase all those reducing products. We need to feel that we are active in the process of losing weight. The purchasing of diet foods makes us feel as though we are indeed doing something.

How to stop playing the game: Recognize that if you eat a can of food containing 200 calories, and have a choice between that and a non-diet food of half the volume but identical in calories, the caloric yield of both is the same. You must ask yourself:

1. Is it really necessary to purchase the diet product?
2. Why am I buying this specific food?
3. Is it really going to help me?

If your answer is that you need more food for less calories while really losing weight, then purchasing a diet food is valid. If, however, you buy the diet food just because it makes you feel that you are dieting successfully, and proceed to consume as much diet food as you would regular food, you wind up with the same amount of binging calories. If this is the outcome, you are truly fooling yourself.

6. The "I Am Going To My Diet Group So It's Okay If I'm Not 100% Good" Game.

How and why we play the game: We faithfully show up at our weekly meeting and confess that we are not following the diet to a "T". We need to feel that as long as we are doing something about our diet—showing up at the weekly meeting—we are truly dieting.

How to stop playing the game: Recognize that the function of the weekly group meeting is sharing your feelings, but that talk does not mean success. Remember the old saying, "Actions speak louder than words." As long as you view your weekly meetings as an aid in dieting, you are safe. One of my own sayings is, "Knowledge is not power. Power is the ability to act upon knowledge."

7. The "I Am So Depressed, Why Bother To Try?" Game.

How and why we play the game: We convince ourselves that while in a depressed state there is absolutely no chance for us to pull ourselves together. We need this excuse in order to give ourselves more time. This is otherwise known as the "grand delay of the inevitable" or "the super cop-out." This game might very well turn into another one of my very favorite sayings: "I can't lose weight until I get my life together, but I can't get my life together until I lose weight." This represents a stalemate, the perfect Catch-22. No movement whatsoever.

Rather than saying, "I do not want to put in the effort at this time that losing weight requires," we say, "I will depend on my depression to give me an excuse." Facing our weakness with that excuse is indeed very difficult. To plug into our depression as the reason for our inability to diet is very easy.

How to stop playing the game: As soon as you recognize that you are looking for an excuse—*Beware!* The more cop-outs you recognize in yourself, the closer you can get to assuming responsibility for your own actions. It is in your awareness of your internal dialogue that you can make changes. Without this awareness there can be no changes.

8. The "Feigned Illness" Game.

How and why we play the game: We give ourselves an excuse to go off our diet ("feed a cold"); or we avoid going into a situation where our being overweight would make us uncomfortable, such as, "I can't go to that beach party because I'm coming down with something."

How to stop playing the game: In avoiding a situation we are in essence protecting ourselves. This has its merits. Protection from wounds is nature's way of avoiding pain. Rather than feigning an illness or giving any other made-up excuse, simply acknowledge that you are not ready. There is nothing wrong with not being ready; hopefully, as long as we are honest with ourselves, others will appreciate it. Another way of looking at a potentially uncomfortable situation is to view it in relation to how good we will make others feel by going, and not always put ourselves in the emotional limelight.

9. The "All Or Nothing" Game.

Why we play the game: We give ourselves an excuse to turn a minor deviation from a diet into an all-out binge: "As long as I've always had one cookie, I might as well finish the box," or, "I've cheated at lunch, so now the whole day is shot"; or, "Since I can't do it all the way, I might as well not do it at all."

How to stop playing the game: Binges come in all sizes. You *can* learn to control the size of the binge to which that first compulsive bite leads. It is far better after having had that first cookie to have five more than to finish the entire box. And, in fact, it is sometimes far better to have those five cookies than to have none at all. It is my feeling that total denial often leads to an all-out binge, whereas the satisfaction of having a few cookies may help to keep us on course.

The games can go on and on and on, ad infinitum.

In conclusion, we all have tapes that keep running through our brains: You have your very own set of dieting game tapes. It would be an interesting exercise for you to follow the format I have used in discovering your own system. Name your game, discover how and why you play it, and decide how you can stop playing it. Here are some additional game titles you may want to fill in yourself:

1. The "It's Too Hard To Diet" Game
2. The "I Will Use A Liquid Diet To Get Me Started" Game
3. The "If I Go Away For A Few Weeks To A Diet Spa It Will Get Me Started" Game
4. The "I Can't Diet At All No Matter How Hard I Try, So I Might As Well Give Up Forever" Game
5. The "I'll Exercise Off That Chocolate Bar" Game
6. The "I Have A Hurt And Have To Make It 'Better' " Game
7. The "I Must Have A Metabolic Problem" Game
8. The "I Can Lose Weight Faster Than You Can" Game

After eleven years of practicing weight counseling I can say with clear conscience that I have never met a patient, barring any medical complications, incapable of losing weight. It is, rather, that the person is unwilling and not fully committed to the project. Many times, however, facing the pain we must overcome in conquering our obesity, we choose to remain with the familiar agony of our weight problem. We now have a choice.

Now that I have exposed you to some of the Alternate's various ways of playing its game, I will show you the many stages that your Alternate goes through, all of which lead to food being put in your mouth. Then, not only will you understand what is happening, but most important, you will have ways to cope and to reach your ultimate goal—that of being thin.

QUESTIONS AND ANSWERS ABOUT *THE BRAND NAME DIET*

What should your goal weight be? You should discard all former charts that indicate what your weight should be according to age, frame and height. According to Dr. Hilde Bruch, a noted psychiatrist who has devoted much time to the subject of obesity, the weight at which a woman functions best and at which she is not unduly fatigued or irritable is her right weight and her biologically meaningful weight. In my opinion, this applies equally to men. If you are 5'6", there is no reason why you should be straitjacketed into a specific goal weight. If you feel and look well at 149 lbs., why is it that, according to authorities, you have failed until such time as you weigh what *they* say you have to weigh? I don't believe in dictatorships, and so I am letting *you* decide what weight you want to attain.

Do you always have to eat breakfast, lunch and dinner? Absolutely not. Here again, the dictators threaten you with "You must have three square meals a day, or else." I feel that you should eat and plan your meals and snacks to be consumed whenever *you* so desire. I am in full agreement with Frederick J. Stare, M.D., Chairman of the department of nutrition at Harvard University, who says that the theory that you need to have three meals a day for a balanced diet is false. The number of times a day you eat is not that important, providing that what you eat in a twenty-four-hour period satisfies your body's needs.

Furthermore, although you do need milk or milk products, it is false that everybody needs at least two cups of milk a day. They can be replaced by ice cream, ice milk, cottage cheese or cheese. On the other hand, if you like skimmed milk, I have provided for you to have it in The Brand Name Diet.

Do you have to have everything that is written in The Brand Name Diet? Will it destroy the diet's chemical balance if you don't? Absolutely not. There is no rhyme or reason why anybody should cram down your throat food that you do not want on a particular day. You need not feed a hunger that is not hungry. Dictators like to dictate, but I'd like to ask any one of them, "Do you sleep exactly seven hours, twenty-nine minutes and four seconds every night?" I would like to ask them if they urinate at precisely 9:30 in the morning, 2:12 in the afternoon, and 8:16 in the evening. I would like to ask them if they have sex at exactly 3:14 in the afternoon on Thursdays, Sundays and Tuesdays. Although they don't specify the time you have to eat breakfast, lunch and dinner, they do demand of you that you mechanize your eating patterns for the sake of re-educating your eating habits.

Skipped meals can lead to overeating at the next meal or between meals; they can result in decreased efficiency, slower mental reactions, and increased muscular fatigue. So it's better not to skip meals regularly. But, I am totally against turning human beings into robots; since it's your body and your mind, you should feed them when *you* feel the need. Just as there are some times when I just feel like going for a walk, and other times when I curl up with a good book, my eating patterns vary too. There are times when I skip breakfast and have a delightful brunch. There are times when I work right through the usual dinner hour without a hunger pang, and at those times I enjoy a late evening feast. Sometimes I skip lunch because I have to; sometimes I do so by choice—and at those times I have a blissful cocktail hour filled with delicious and nutritious foods. I am free to be me, and I want you to keep your freedom to be you.

Do you like the physical sensation of a full stomach? If your answer is yes, we'll fill it to the brim. If your answer is no, and you prefer light meals, you will be able to do so. "I eat almost every hour on the hour, and sometimes feel miserable if I can't do so. Is that wrong? Will it keep me from losing weight?" If you feel happy nibbling away, go right ahead. It can do you no harm but, quite the contrary, much good—because you will NOT be miserable. If you basically follow a diet on which you are meant to lose weight, it does not matter how many meals or snacks you make out of it.

THE NEVERS

Remember, I have no "don'ts," "can'ts," "musts" and "always," but I do have three important "nevers."

Never think, if you should occasionally slip up, that you are *cheating*. "Cheating" is defined in a leading dictionary as "one who or that which deceives or defrauds; an impostor or imposture." The synonym "impostor" is "one who imposes upon others for the purpose of deception; a pretender."

This most ugly word—cheating—which has been so widely used by my colleagues, is one of the most vile accusations that I can think of. Imagine calling somebody a fraud because he or she might have had a bad day and might have nibbled at a cookie. Imagine being given a 6-ounce portion of steak and being labelled an impostor just for having one more tiny piece. I feel angry when I recall that I was once one of those almighty lecturers who pointed the finger at someone who had worked so much and had fought so hard, and reduced that person to a "cheat"—just because they had an emotional crisis—a sick child, perhaps, or a flunked exam—that resulted in a mere half-pound gain.

Another *Never* is that damaging word *guilt*. Granted that you are responsbile for slipping off your diet, but the word "guilty" should be erased from your vocabulary forever in connection with food. Instead, after the food has been eaten, just think, "It happened and it is a learning experience for the future." You cannot do anything about the minute behind you, so why bother to dwell on it? The minute in front of you is *hope*.

The last *Never* is: Never emphasize the negative; always emphasize the positive. Stop beating yourself on the head. Stop kicking yourself around. Stop cursing at yourself. What good is it? In the past you have been abused, accused, and treated like some kind of criminal. You felt like a cheat because you were told you were a cheat. That's all over.

Trying is never failing.

METHODS OF TEACHING

No two people are capable of losing weight in exactly the same way, and since conquering the weight problem is an educational process, we must approach it with flexibility. It is incongruous that most of those who offer dieting help claim that only their way will solve *everyone's* problem. Your weight problem will be solved—but with *The Brand Name Diet* you will be the one in charge of your own decision making.

IX

Techniques for Coping With Your Foods and Feelings

Here are some tools that will help you deal with your weight problems. My purpose in giving you these techniques is to enable you to become more aware of your eating behavior and to modify it by knowing just where you are in every given situation. Furthermore, you will be able to recognize the various stages of your own patterns and hence be able to cope with them.

The techniques are:

1. Binge Awarnesss
2. The Pre-Binge State
3. The Post-Binge State (Foods and Feeling Memory Bank)
4. Plateau Coping
5. Portion Control
6. Flexible Eating Behavior

BINGE AWARENESS

Let's examine the ways in which the Alternate operates. One of the more terrifying aspects of the overeating syndrome is the *binge*. The dictionary definition of *binge* is "spree," and *spree* is defined as "a lively frolic." However, to the compulsive overeater, there is seldom anything lively or frolicsome about a binge or its aftermath. A more relevant definition is needed. For our purposes, a binge may be defined as a period of compulsive eating of foods that cause weight gain (mostly carbohydrates and fats). Binges vary in intensity and type:

1. The most terrifying binge is the one we find ourselves in without knowing how we got there. Our "blanking out" as we enter the binge is a defense mechanism to protect us from the stark reality of what we are doing to ourselves. This tuning out of our emotions is a subject that I consider of great importance in the understanding of bingeing behavior. We must at all times try to raise our level of consciousness regarding our eating behavior. This gives us the opportunity to make the decision whether or not we wish to impose any controls. When we "tune out" we relinquish this power to make decisions.

2. The planned binge is somewhat less terrifying, if only because we know it is coming. The binge is first created in our minds. We may be aroused by passing a bakery for instance. The senses involved here are:

   a. *Vision.* The sight of a plump light brown doughnut with a thick layer of chocolate frosting stimulates a desire.

   b. *Smell.* The soft, sweet aromas arouse our olfactory sense.

   c. *Imagination.* We create in our minds what it would be like to hold the doughnut in our hand, to bite into its doughy sweet consistency, to savour its scrumptious flavor, and BINGO!—we are turned on. We are so aroused that eating it seems to be a MUST! Somehow while purchasing that one doughnut, we buy two or three more, knowing very well from past experience that one lonely doughnut will just act as a tease, and that we will reason since we are going off our diets anyhow, we might as well really enjoy it (The All or Nothing Game).

d. *Taste.* We may be offered a cookie at the office, and asked for our instant opinion. It is offered so quickly that neither vision, smell nor imagination has been aroused. The focal point in our excitement is now our mouth—and BINGO—we are turned on! Our imagination soon takes over again and we feel we must re-create that pleasure. Since it is unlikely that we can attack all the cookies to be shared by our co-workers, we begin to become restless and anxious for the business day to end. Although we may be going about our duties on a conscious level, our Alternate is very actively planning where it is going to go at 5 P.M. and what it is going to buy.

THE PRE-BINGE STATE

The Pre-Binge State is our own built-in warning system, much as a yellow flashing light at an intersection warns us to slow down because of possible danger ahead. It is that period of time between being turned on to the idea of food and actually consuming it. The Pre-Binge State can last for many hours or for as little as a fraction of a second. For instance, looking back at the situation of the cookie being offered in the office, the Pre-Binge State lasted until the end of the working day—several hours. However, if we're in the kitchen, it takes only a split second to reach into the cookie jar.

I have talked about the various stimuli connected with food (vision, smell, imagination and taste). Everybody reacts to these physical stimuli in pretty much the same way. However, the emotional factors that lead to the Pre-Binge State are much more individualized.

We are emotional eaters and recognize that fact, but the recognition is not the solution. It is only the first step toward coping.

For example, you have been unjustly fired or denied a promotion. You are angry, hurt and depressed. You have an emotional "gap." In examining this so far, there is nothing you can do to ameliorate the situation. Your natural tendency is to seek comfort, and your problem is that you have learned to seek comfort in food. So you have an all-out binge, and are left with:

a. The employment situation unchanged
b. Anger, hurt and depression
c. An added problem, that of remorse and extra weight

The binge was instantaneous comfort and escape. Pleasure was, in fact, felt for the duration of the binge—but you are now left with hours of pain. Is it worth it? At times there is nothing you can or want to do to avert a binge. This is very normal.

The techniques I am describing lessen the severity of your bingeing and reduce its frequency, while not completely stripping you of your traditional means of comfort. If you try to use these methods you should be very, very tolerant and patient with yourself at the beginning. Mistakes are to be expected in any learning process in any area of life.

What To Do While In The Pre-Binge State—
The Three Stages

STAGE 1: At this stage, the Pre-Binge State is recognized, confronted and accepted. You will recognize it because you feel a tremendous tension within your mind that pulls your thoughts to food. At this time, you must question why you are feeling this way. If possible, try to solve the problem that has led you to the Pre-Binge State. If there is no way of solving the problem, you can choose to direct your thoughts away from an oncoming binge. Try deep breathing exercises, slowly massaging your temples while visualizing a deserted tropical beach setting. Or try going for a very brisk five minute walk. You can develop your own methods for distracting your mind from food.

STAGE 2: If using behavioral and psychological tools such as those cited above do not work, the goalization technique might be very helpful. "Goalization" is deep concentration on either the reason why you want to lose weight or the reason you have chosen not to remain overweight. You may find that by nibbling on assorted low-calorie vegetables or drinking a cup of hot broth you will avoid the consumption of high calorie foods. Losing weight must become a stronger desire than that of wanting to binge.

Your most important tool is *time:* time to think about why you want to lose weight; time to think about whether the food will make the problem go away; time to think about the feeling of satisfaction you'll get from being able to control your Alternate; time to think about what is causing the tension or anxiety that has put you into the Pre-Binge State. Perhaps you cannot change the situation that has brought you into the Pre-Binge State. If not, you *can* still change your reaction to that situation.

STAGE 3: This is the delicious state of euphoria that you've earned by your perseverance in plowing through the stages necessary to avoid the binge. Another step closer to your goal of mastering self-control.

THE POST-BINGE STATE

Foods and Feelings Memory Bank

When we binge we eat *foods* and then have *feelings*. The *foods* are usually delicious carbohydrates (starches and sugars); the *feelings* are usually negative. We can make use of this Post-Binge State by storing it in our "Foods and Feelings Memory Bank."

Two of the most common reactions we find we have had after a binge are:

1. To promptly try to block out all of our negative feelings connected with the binge: "It really wasn't so much after all;" "I had to do it and it was good that I got it out of my system;" "I don't have to be concerned because from now on I'm going to go straight!"
2. To feed on the negative feelings that the binge produces in us. These in turn give us an out for another binge: "Well, this just proves once again that I have no will power—so there's no use in fighting it"; "I am so depressed and I feel so rotten because of what I've done, I might as well keep bingeing—what's the use?"; "This last binge has proved to me that I'll never make it."

You must recognize that by avoiding your feelings or by drowning yourself in guilt and defeatism, you can make no progress.

How You Can Use The Post-Binge State
To Your Advantage

A Foods and Feelings Memory Bank is a place in which to store the binge and its aftermath for future motivation and reference. This is how it works:

Next time a binge approaches, go to your Foods and Feelings Memory Bank and pull out the last binge. Examine what it did for you and how you felt about it. Do you want to experience those feelings again? Do you want to pay the price again? Can you in all honesty say that the food was really that satisfying? Can you remember saying to yourself, "I hope this never happens again"? This is making use of a past food event as a source of motivation for coping with a present situation.

Sometimes looking into the future and thinking why you want to lose weight doesn't have enough of a punch. But many times looking into the past can provide that needed jolt.

When about to binge, we capitalize on whatever positive association we can make with food. We remember the smell, the taste and texture. This is called the *Food Feeling*. What we don't, or do not want to, remember as an association with that food is the negative feelings we had *after* we binged on it the last time. We are pleasure seekers and therefore conveniently forget the aspects of a past event that caused us discomfort. If we allow ourselves only to remember the delicious aspects of the binge, we are bound to want to recreate its pleasure.

Our Foods and Feelings Memory Bank can be used as a working tool to help us avoid the binge either by remembering the satisfaction we derived from avoiding our last binge, or remembering the agitation and depression that it caused.

Our memory can be one of our most important tools, if we learn to cultivate it.

PLATEAU COPING

There are occasions in any successful diet when, despite all our efforts, our weight remains the same for a period of time. If we are not prepared for this, it can be a very frustrating and demoralizing experience. We are apt to give up because we equate dieting with continuous weight loss, and forget that dieting can also be weight maintaining. We must learn to appreciate our emotional growth as well as our physical weight loss. Exercising emotional control without deriving a weight loss can be regarded as a satisfying experience. If we were to exercise no control we would, in all probability, gain.

From a clinical point of view, there is an explanation for the plateau which is most often overlooked. It has been scientifically proven that the more you weigh, the more calories you need to maintain that weight. The exact same diet that would cause a 275-pound person to lose weight could quite easily cause someone weighing 175 pounds to gain. As your weight decreases, the calorie intake you need to maintain it decreases, and therefore the intake needed to continue your weight loss also decreases. You may have to adjust your diet so that the plateau period is shortened.

When you reach a plateau, I suggest that:

a. Although you may feel it is the end of the world and that you are working in vain, it is one of those uncomfortable states that you must plow through.
b. You take a look at your diet and see how it compares to the way you were eating when you first started losing

weight. If your diet is very much the same, cut back a little and see what happens (specific suggestions appear later).

c. If you cut back and still nothing happens, you may have to ride it out and rely on what you have already accomplished to lessen the frustration.

If you get into a habit of periodically writing down everything you eat and drink during a day, it will help you make comparisons and adjustments later on.

PORTION CONTROL

You and I know from past experience how painful and difficult it is to take only three or four spoonfuls of ice cream from a half-gallon container. The remaining ice cream haunts us, and our Alternate, having had its appetite whetted, usually drives us to want to consume all of it. The reason we feel the few spoonfuls represent such a small amount is that in comparison to what remains, our portion looks like next to nothing. That firm, hard ice-cream square has been slightly dented by our spoon, and many times our Alternate proceeds to its favorite ice-cream game.

Have you ever run your spoon around the four sides of the carton and then gingerly made those edges smooth again so that there were no gaping holes for anyone to detect? Have you ever seen yourself slowly, meticulously lowering the amount in the carton, when you knew your Alternate was really fooling you? The following experience will clearly define what I am talking about:

A 3-ounce portion of ice cream from a half-gallon container looks absurd. A 3-ounce portion from a quart looks a little better, but still like a tease. A 3-ounce portion from a pint starts to look like something, but the temptation to have more is still too strong. A 3-ounce portion from a half-pint is something, but the Alternate's instinct to have just a tiny bit more is overpowering. A 3-ounce portion from a three-ounce Dixie Cup *is* the entire container!

The Alternate derives great satisfaction from finishing things. If, therefore, we pre-control the portion we are going to have (and by the way, I give you real ice cream in Dixie Cups and prepackaged ice-cream bars in *The Brand Name Diet*), the Alternate is automatically controlled.

In this way we ensure that we are not only nutritionally well fed, but also emotionally well fed. That is, we feed our Alternate. Since the Alternate can get wild when given large quantities and told it can only have a tiny amount, we have found a way to feed the Alternate in a controlled situation. This is *portion control.*

If you put a fried egg on a meat platter, it gets lost on that great span of china, and looks very small and lonely. You react to that situation by feeling that you're having practically nothing. Your Alternate hates that, and starts bugging you. Now put that same fried egg on a bread and butter dish, and the Alternate becomes ecstatic as it sees the "large" portion. I am not proposing that you eat your food from dollhouse china, but the size of the plate can calm the Alternate.

There are times when our Alternate cannot stand the idea of counting, weighing or measuring its treats. It flies into a rage because it wants the whole thing from start to finish. I have provided an entire package of popped corn in *The Brand Name Diet*. The package is great to take to the movies, to have on a picnic or just to munch on while watching television. This is the secret to portion control. The foods you believe to be dangerous villains because you have been taught to think that way are really your friends when their amount is controlled. You won't believe that in just a few short weeks you will be eating doughnuts, popped corn, cake, crackers and cookies while you lose weight. The secret is *portion control*.

The concept of portion control is to keep you and your Alternate happy in a controlled way by having prepackaged items that can be eaten from start to finish without ever suffering again that big box on your lap, which you and I know is difficult to deal with. You will find that throughout *The Brand Name Diet*, foods that used to haunt you and cause a weight gain are now given to you in a fashion that will delight you and cause a weight loss.

That old saying "It's not what you eat, it's how much you eat," is accurate—*except* that no one has ever taken your Alternate into consideration in controlling how much. Now you have—for the rest of your life—*portion control*, which as you will learn, does not feel like deprivation. Just the opposite. It feels like freedom.

FLEXIBLE EATING BEHAVIOR

One of the major problems of overeating is the ready availability of food. At one of the larger universities this problem has been studied in a program where patients live under controlled conditions. They are not permitted to leave the premises and their meals are served to them in a regimented fashion. There is no access to foods other than what is served.

Along with this diet control, psychological counseling is given in conjunction with behavior modification. The treatment is an outstanding success for those who stay on the premises. The problems arise when the patients return to their normal, uncontrolled environment. Although studies have shown a good percentage of people "surviving" on the outside, we are concerned with those who have a rebound syndrome.

THE BRAND NAME DIET

I believe that we must learn to "fit our diet into our life, not our life into our diet." We do not live in cocoons; life is a series of unexpected events.

For instance, there is a difference between making a phone call and receiving one. When we place a call we know whom we are calling and why. When our phone rings, we have no idea who it might be and we are unprepared—caught off guard. This unexpected feeling occurs in many situations regarding dieting: There is no surprise element to be dealt with when we plan and prepare our own meals. A dinner invitation, however, brings us face to face with the unexpected. If we only learn to cope with controlled situations, we are powerless to deal with the unexpected—and the unexpected is our Alternate's playground.

One of the ways in which we can deal with an unexpected situation is to turn it into a facsimile of a situation that is controlled. For example, a woman I was counseling had been abstaining from one of her favorite treats, chocolate bars, for a considerable period. She found that she was beginning to become obsessed with thoughts of chocolate bars. This obsession reached its peak when she woke in the middle of one night from a very vivid dream of eating chocolate bars. She was afraid she was on the verge of a major binge. She placed a call to us the following morning, in desperate need of advice.

Our discussion of the situation led to the following experimental strategy: She was to buy one chocolate bar during her lunch break, and take it back to her office. In this controlled environment she would be able to consume only this one candy bar, without immediate access to more. She would do this in order to:

a. See if the taste of chocolate would be sufficient to satisfy her craving

b. See if one chocolate bar could now satisfy her as much as
several used to

At the conclusion of her experiment, she found that the
one bar gave her enough satisfaction. She ate the candy
slowly (knowing it was the only one available), taking the
time to enjoy its taste, aroma and texture. The time that
elapsed while she ate this one candy bar was approximately
the same as she had previously taken to gobble down five or
six. The pleasure of consuming the five or six bars had been
offset by the weight gain it produced, but the equal pleasure
of consuming the one bar was enhanced by the weight loss
attained that week!

The concept of having controlled pleasures in dieting, and
feeling the freedom of total choice with the application of
portion control, places a new value on food itself. There is
virtually no food that need be denied the dieter, provided
only that control is exercised with regard to quantity and
frequency.

Moderation is the key to success—abuse is the key to obesity. If
you are convinced that you can never have this kind of control, think again. Learning portion control is like any other
learning experience: It takes time and practice. Sometimes
you don't make it; you fall back and binge. But each time
you *do* make it gives you strength for the next time. A few
successes here and there lead to more frequent successes.

The watchword is *time*. Your Alternate has spent a long
time building up your destructive eating patterns, and it will
take time to change them into constructive ones. Be patient
with yourself.

X

The Food Link Between
Parent and Child

In raising children, parents take on a vast array of responsibilities, and hopefully, after growing up, the children will be happy, productive, emotionally and physically healthy human beings. One of the absolute necessities on the part of the parent is to feed the child.

Feeding a child is instinctive on the part of the mother and father. If a baby is wailing and both parents have checked for clean diapers and open safety pins, and everything checks out all right, the next thing that jumps into their minds is, "Oh my gosh, the baby must be hungry." There are some pediatricians who believe that a baby should not be put on a specific feeding schedule during infancy, and there are others who insist that the parents nourish their child according to the clock.

I don't remember whether as a baby I cried because I was

hungry, because I wanted to be held, because I was mad that I couldn't turn over in my crib, or just for the sake of crying. The line of communication between myself and my parents was either a coo and a smile or a loud cry with a red face. I don't think that it can be scientifically proved exactly why a baby cries at any given moment. I do know from the experience of raising my own child and of having been exposed to training in pediatrics that a bottle or a breast can do wonders.

If I could for a few days become a baby, of all the activities available to me, such as being dressed, bathed, powdered, rocked, etc., I think I would choose feeding as my first choice. Why? First of all, I would have to be held and would be very close to a warm body. Then my sucking instinct would be taken care of by the sensation of the nipple. Next I would feel a warm, rather sweet liquid in my mouth, and my tummy would happily fill up. In between, my back would be gently rubbed so that I could burp. I would be handled with tender loving care as I was put down after my feeding.

Let us assume for a moment that I am a superintelligent infant. I quickly figure out that all I have to do is scream my head off, and my parents, at my command, will reenact the link of love and food. This is purely hypothetical, but to this day I associate eating with ingesting pleasure, warmth, cuddliness, satisfaction, security, and deriving tremendous oral gratification.

It is not, however, the infancy stage which I am so concerned about. It is the period of time when a child is able to verbalize its desires and needs. Since we as parents learn to pacify an infant with food, we then continue to use food as a means of quieting a child. How many times have you been in a store and seen a toddler crying while sitting in its carriage? From the parents' point of view there is nothing like placing a cookie in the baby's hand. This gives parents a few moments of respite from the crying, until the cookie has either been eaten or accidentally—or intentionally— dropped, and the cycle repeats itself. Parent quiets child with food.

Now the parent, as the child grows older, starts to use food as a means of discipline or motivation. It is quite common during the toilet training period that, if the child successfully completes its mission on the toilet, and not in its pants, it is rewarded with some treat—invariably some form of starch or sugar. In giving this goodie for a successful visit to the bathroom, the parent tries to motivate the child by saying, "Next time you go potty, you'll get a lollipop."

Let us assume again, for a moment, that I am a superbrainy kid. I quickly figure out that all I have to do to get that yummy lollipop is to hold in my urine and go potty every fifteen minutes. To my parent's delight, I am on my way to being toilet trained. To my delight, I am on my way to Lollipop Land. But neither my parents nor I understand that this kind of motivation—giving a treat for an accomplishment—is going to create a possible emotional problem in connection with food.

Let us further examine food and its role in the relationship between parent and child. Food is a great instrument of the parent.

PARENT TO CHILD:

1. "Since you have misbehaved, you will have to go to bed without supper." Here, the parent is depriving the child of food as a means of *punishment*.
2. "If you behave yourself and don't cry when the doctor gives you an injection, I promise that I will buy you your

very favorite ice cream." Here, the parent is using food as a means of a *bribe*.

3. "I am so delighted with your report card that I will let you have two desserts tonight." Here, the parent is using food as a means of *reward*.

4. "I am so sorry that your team lost the ball game. Go into the kitchen and cut yourself a nice piece of chocolate cake and have a glass of milk. It'll make you feel better." Here, the parent is using food as a means of *consolation*.

5. "Since you're home sick today and you're really not feeling well, I prepared some yummy chocolate pudding and bought your favorite marshmallow cookies." Here the parent is using food as a means of *comfort*.

6. "I know what it's like to lose a friend and how terrible you feel. I'll make you a homemade hot fudge sundae— it'll help the tears go away." Here the parent is using food as an *emotional pain reliever*.

There are many ways of disciplining, motivating, soothing, comforting, showing disapproval, praising a child, etc. Food must *never, never, never* be used as a *tool*. Food should be presented to the child as a source of nutrition which is good to eat and which leads to a sound body and mind. Granted that there are times, such as the special occasion of a birthday party or other exciting events, when foods that are starchy and sweet are presented to the child. I have never known anyone to become fat from celebrating such an occasion using moderation. It is those in-between times that I am talking about.

I specifically used carbohydrates in the above examples only to dramatize the fact that sweets and starches play such a vital role in the overweight problem that you and I face today. As a matter of fact, the carbohydrate problem goes even deeper than being used as a tool of behavior. Do you remember your parents telling you that you had to finish your vegetables before you could eat your dessert? That is why desserts have become a special problem for you. You were taught that they were very special foods, and perhaps vegetables and salads were negatively emphasized as a means of getting to that crowning glory of the meal, the dessert.

Food must always be neutral territory.

CARBOHYDRATES FROM INFANCY ON

Invariably, after a baby is born, the first source of nutrition to reach its mouth is slightly sweetened water. The very next source of nutrition is either mother's milk or formula. Both contain a form of sugar necessary for the physiological well being of the infant. So far so good; the carbohydrate problem begins when the child starts eating baby food.

You will discover, to your surprise, how vital a role the baby food manufacturers, and parents, play in actually developing your child's special attachment for *sweets* and *starches*. Almost every baby food manufacturer used to add sugar to vegetables, and additional sugar to its fruit products. If a baby is fed sweetened carrots and squash, its palate becomes conditioned to those foods having a sweet taste. As a result, the child starts developing a food problem when given "grown-up foods." The child, having been trained on sweetened baby foods, turns away from carrots and squash presented in an unsweetened state. (That is not always the case; there are many, many children who, having been fed baby food, grow up eating a vast array of vegetables without any difficulty. They have escaped our problem because, for some reason or another, their emotional and physiological makeup is different.)

Often, parents add to the baby-food problem in the way they feed their children. I have seen countless mothers feed their children a meal by giving them a teaspoonful of sweet applesauce right after or just before a spoonful of cereal. Sometimes when the parent is faced with a finicky eater, the parent will carefully fill half the spoon with applesauce and half with vegetable. Conceivably the child will think of food as always having a sweet taste. Therefore, when the child is later introduced to bits of meat and vegetable, the child automatically refuses them because something is missing. Parents who are concerned about their children drinking milk will often sweeten it with cherry or chocolate syrup. Children who refuse to eat cut-up fresh fruit will often have a parent sprinkle some sugar on it.

I do not propose that all of us who are fat have this problem because of our excessive sugar intake during childhood. Many of you have been fat since childhood, many of you developed a problem during your teenage years, many of you developed a problem during your pregnancy or after childbirth, and many of you found yourself overweight well after you were into your middle adult years. Childhood eating habits are not the only reason for an overweight problem in later years. Many children with poor eating experiences later develop into slim adults with no trace of an overeating problem. But there are studies that show that the way a child is fed can create problems with food later in life.

The entire dental and medical professions agree that Americans have too much sugar in their diets. It is quick and easy to hand a child some cookies for a snack because no work is required on the part of the parent. But giving an apple to a child also requires no work, and nutritionally the apple far outweighs the cookies. It is so simple to put some marshmallows in a dish, but it is also simple to peel an orange. If children are taught to equate between-meal snack foods with carbohydrates, that equation becomes a set way of dealing with food in later years.

Again, there are many, many people who are very healthy and who have a few cookies for an afternoon snack. You must again understand that I am only concerned with *you*. You are the one who does not know how to have only a few cookies. You seem to need more, and that's the problem I'm concerned with.

I cannot take you back to your childhood and show your parents where they might have veered you in the wrong direction in connection with food. But your children and grandchildren may be spared a possible overweight problem if you learn to undo the "excessive intake of carbohydrates" syndrome.

A stark example about a food we love so much will clearly explain how a taste reaction to a food is ingrained. For years and years you have delighted in eating sweet chocolate. It is not only the chocolate taste that you like, but the fact that it's sweet. If you were to eat some unsweetened baking chocolate, the chocolate taste would still be there, but the sweetness would be missing. You would then be turned off to the baking chocolate, but *only* because the sweetness is missing. By the same token, if a baby is fed sweetened string beans, you can clearly comprehend why an unsweetened string bean poses an eating problem.

In conclusion, I am not against carbohydrates being an integral part of a daily diet. But I am strongly opposed to carbohydrates being used either as "food foolers" or the only source of snacks. As a matter of fact, when I am helping children or adolescents with overweight problems, I always have a conference, if possible—with *both parents*.

It is very difficult to help an obese child whose brothers or sisters have no weight problems. The siblings have free access to the kitchen without adding extra pounds. The obese child also wants to have freedom in the kitchen. I am totally against depriving other family members of the foods that create problems for the obese child, as I am totally opposed to just telling the child, "You have a weight problem and you are not allowed in the kitchen." I have solved this dilemma for many parents and children, having first introduced the following concept in an elementary school.

The obese child was given a very special, large food container with his or her name on it, to be kept in the refrigerator. It was the parent's responsibility to keep that special box filled with low-calorie vegetables, a few cookies, a few slices of cheese, and a few very thin pretzel sticks. During the initial counseling session with the child, he or she was told that there was a very special box in the refrigerator to which he or she had access whenever it was snack time. The box was to be filled only once a day by the parent and it was the child's decision either to eat its contents all at one time or to take food from it until the box was empty.

Most of the children I work with choose to go to their very special box at several intervals. They say that they feel like one of the gang because now they can always go into the kitchen and there is always something to eat. These children are losing weight and are physically very healthy. But just as important, they are emotionally happy because they do not feel deprived of "refrigerator rights" when they see their siblings marching in and out of the kitchen.

There are some parents who believe in three square meals a day, and that's that. They enforce rigidity on their children while they are content to have their mid-morning coffee break, before-dinner cocktail, and snack before bedtime. Children are no less human than adults, and imposing such rigid meal controls may later cause the child to rebel: "Now

I can eat when I damn well feel like it." This new attitude can cause obesity.

There is absolutely no harm in snacking, but there is potential harm in what and how much is given.